THE *STRANDS* OF SPEECH AND LANGUAGE THERAPY

WEAVING A THERAPY PLAN FOR NEUROREHABILITATION

Katy James, Jacqueline McIntosh, Nicole Charles, Brenda Lyons & Beverley Leach

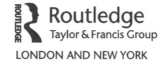

Routledge
Taylor & Francis Group

LONDON AND NEW YORK

First published 2011 by Speechmark Publishing Ltd.

2 Park Square, Milton Park, Abingdon, Oxfordshire OX14 4RN
52 Vanderbilt Avenue, New York, NY 10017

Routledge is an imprint of the Taylor & Francis Group, an informa business -

First issued in paperback 2018

British Library cataloguing in publication data
A catalogue record for this book is available from the British Library.

ISBN 978-1-138-43425-7 (hbk)
ISBN 978-0-86388-815-1 (pbk)

Contents

Acknowledgements

We would like to thank our colleagues who have been members of the Speech and Language Therapy team at different times during the compilation of this book. They have provided us with support in different ways – initial planting of seeds, discussion of ideas, listening, 'editing', case discussions, and taking on board our 'Strands' philosophy and integrating it into their work. Particular mention goes to Claire Farrington-Douglas, Vicky Lack and Annie Voullaire.

We would also like to thank members of the team at The Wolfson Neurorehabilitation Centre, and especially our patients, who are at the centre of our work.

Introduction

Neurorehabilitation is a fairly young field that continues to grow and develop as more research is conducted. It is well recognised in the literature that there are a number of elements that should be seen as having more or less equal status and importance in aphasia rehabilitation. Code & Muller (1989), and more recently Kagan *et al* (2008), describe in detail the importance of essential perspectives that must be considered by therapists when assessing and developing their therapeutic approach with individuals presenting with aphasia:

1 linguistic methodology

2 non-verbal communication

3 neurology and neuropsychological processing

4 psychosocial factors

5 behavioural methodology

6 evaluation, review and modification – a hypothesis testing approach.

To outline, these authors state that a therapeutic programme should have its foundations in the linguistic, non-verbal, neurological and neuropsychological perspectives of the patient's difficulties, and the therapist should utilise a systematic behavioural strategy for therapy presentation, while considering the patient's psychosocial state and requirements (Code & Muller, 1989). Furthermore, there should be ongoing and consistent evaluation of the patient's response to therapy using hypotheses and modification of treatment.

These six perspectives have formed the foundation of our Speech and Language Therapy (SLT) service delivery at the Wolfson Neurorehabilitation Centre. We work with individuals presenting with acquired communication disorders that can result from brain injury (for example aphasia, cognitive-communication disorder, dysarthria, apraxia). Over time, we have become aware that our philosophy and vision have continued to grow, considering Code & Muller's six perspectives as we work. We feel strongly that these are not aphasia-specific perspectives, but are relevant to all those whose journey leads them to experience communication disability stemming from neurological injury, and should be applied during our SLT provision in inpatient neurorehabilitation. Furthermore, as our knowledge and experience have grown, we have identified and placed great importance on certain elements that we feel must be integral to therapy if we are to support an individual and their significant others along their rehabilitation pathway. Recent articles in *Aphasiology* further illustrate the wide-ranging role of the speech and language therapist, covering topics from lexical retrieval and semantic knowledge through to accessible public transport.

We are very fortunate to work as a small, close and proactive SLT team who share the same vision for working with those with neurodisability. We have seen the importance of taking time to reflect on our service, our therapy achievements and challenges, and user feedback. From this began a small in-house project reviewing recent cases to explore and document our vision and philosophy. This project quickly blossomed to what has become known affectionately to us as our 'Strands'. It was found that within SLT input there were consistent themes and principles for how those themes were approached. We envisaged each area of input as a 'strand' of therapy and used the analogy of a knitted scarf (Figure 1 overleaf) – the therapy plan – made up of various coloured strands, each strand representing an element of our input: assessment and feedback, goal planning, specific individualised treatment, education, friends and family, and psychosocial adjustment.

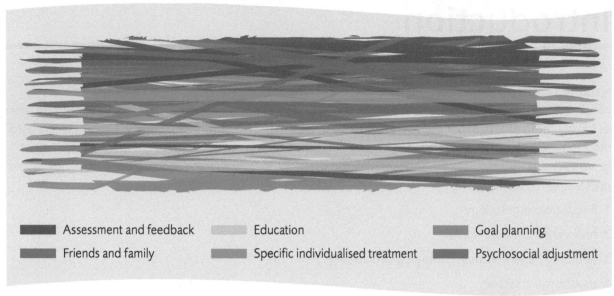

Assessment and feedback Education Goal planning

Friends and family Specific individualised treatment Psychosocial adjustment

Figure 1 The strands of therapy woven into a therapy plan

Code & Muller (1989) refer to the more or less equal status of their six perspectives, and while we agree with this to a degree, we have also found that the 'scarf' is more of a dynamic entity; certain strands may make up a greater proportion of the scarf at various times during the period of SLT involvement, depending on need and timing. We see each client's journey through their brain injury as a long scarf. At certain times in the journey, one colour may be more prevalent than another, but over time each colour should be represented. The client's stay at the rehabilitation centre is just one small part of the longer scarf and so the strands we work on should be considered in the light of what comes before, in the acute stage, and after, in community therapy.

Years of developing an SLT service in response to clients' needs and research developments have resulted in tailor-made intervention programmes, unique to each individual. This makes it difficult for newly qualified therapists and students to grasp what therapy approaches to consider and how to prioritise among them. We have to balance patients' goals, meeting our professional obligations and the demands of working in a multidisciplinary team. We recognise that we are fortunate to have the luxury of working intensively with our patients and the flexibility to provide a range of therapy options such as one to one, groups, multidisciplinary joint sessions, working with family and friends and community-based sessions.

It is the purpose of this text to detail the strands, to illustrate in a user-friendly way how each strand relates to therapy and to give some practical ideas of how we work within each strand at the Wolfson. Each chapter begins with the guiding principles and evidence base that have developed from team discussions about our vision and philosophy, and from literature review, and that form the basis of each strand's rationale. Following on from that are examples of 'what we do'. We have included one case study ('John') which runs through the text to outline a real-life example of each of the strands, and then a further case example for each individual strand. Colour coding illustrates the strand to which it refers. It is hoped that readers will take the time to view the entire text, seeing the scarf in the way we do: as intertwined strands, each strand needed to make up the whole. We also hope this text can be used as a reference and workbook when therapists need ideas for certain strands of their input at various points along the patient's journey.

We have included a CD-Rom with this book containing a number of resources that we use on a regular basis at the Wolfson Centre. These include patient-related information and advice sheets, and service proformas such as a relationships and conversations questionnaire and group documentation sheets. Our aim is for the reader to use them as needed, either directly as templates, or using the ideas and amending them to the individual setting and patients' specific needs (as we would advocate particularly with the patient information sheets).

1 Assessment and feedback

For patients admitted to the multidisciplinary rehabilitation unit, assessment should be multidimensional and wide-ranging to enable appropriate planning. Assessment is an important dimension to guide differential diagnosis and determine the needs level of the patient, and is a core aspect of specific individualised treatment planning. Done thoroughly, it enables us to formulate initial hypotheses and establish the process of collecting evidence for change. Assessment is also an essential strand of the service within an expert centre; the role of assessment may be as much to inform others (for example the patient, community team colleagues) as to inform those working in the centre.

Guiding principles

Underpinned by theory and keeping abreast of new learning

Theoretical models, neurological and linguistic, are seen to underpin assessment. At the Wolfson we have a philosophy of not 'throwing the baby out with the bathwater' and so make use of access to our neurology colleagues and brain scans to guide us in the initial stages of information gathering. We make reference to the specific neurology, that is, the site and location of the individual's brain injury, to guide us as to the expected communication breakdown. For example, when presented with a diagnosis of brainstem injury we might expect dysarthria; with anoxic brain injury we would perhaps expect a diffuse cognitive-communication disorder; with a right middle cerebral artery infarct we might expect both of those plus more specific problems with affect and non-verbal abilities.

However, we must be aware that lesion site is only ground-clearing information and will not give us the full picture of communication breakdown; considering the neurology alone is insufficient to formulate our hypotheses about the details of communication breakdown. The limitations of attempting to diagnose and describe communication disorders based on lesion site alone can be seen from the emerging evidence that lesions in diverse brain areas can result in similar communication impairments. Thalamic aphasia has long been described, and other subcortical linguistic impairments have been identified more recently. In a review paper written in 1994, Kennedy & Murdoch challenge the fact that language is only represented in the cortex. They discuss the extralinguistic functions of the thalamus and suggest that intervention programmes could be devised on the basis of a detailed description of the patient's communication abilities. Paquier & Mariën (2005) have discussed evidence that implicates the cerebellum in diverse higher cognitive functions such as language. As our understanding of brain injury and communication difficulties increases, it seems that damage to any part of the brain may result in communication changes related to linguistics, cognition or information processing.

It is very important then for speech and language therapists to have a means of assessing and diagnosing communication impairment. It has been identified that in some areas these disorders are currently going untreated (Brady *et al*, 2003). Appropriate treatment is reliant on an accurate understanding of the cause of a client's difficulties. This is well understood in aphasia where models of language processing can identify exactly where in the word retrieval system there is a breakdown (Ellis & Young, 1988). In the context of a cognitive-communication disorder these models are not helpful since word-finding difficulties in these cases may be linked to higher-level skills such as initiation or attention control.

Viewing aphasia as primarily a language disorder has, for many years, informed our assessment and consequential therapy, but more recently recognition, as described above, of the co-occurrence of other cognitive disorders has impacted on the approach we take. This has led us to recognise the need to assess the cognitive linguistic breakdown. Published assessment tools such as Mount Wilga High Level Language Assessment and the Measure of Cognitive-Linguistic Abilities (MCLA) are available (see the Appendix for details of formal and informal assessment tools), but with this recognition has come a burgeoning of new kinds of cognitive-communication disorder and links to traditional views of communication breakdown following brain injury. Frankel *et al* (2007) provide a useful illustration of a woman with aphasia *and* executive difficulties and endeavour to describe what the therapist needs to consider in the assessment and treatment. Evidence of this broadening clinical focus was discussed at the American Speech and Hearing Association annual conference (2005, quoted in Milman *et al*, 2008). It was stated that clinicians working in rehabilitation in the USA reported that a larger proportion of SLT services were directed towards cognitive-communication disorder (32 per cent) than to aphasia (22 per cent). Current ongoing research suggests that approximately 50 per cent of all stroke unit admissions present with some features of cognitive-communication disorder (McIntosh *et al*, 2010).

However, theory must also consider the information the patient brings. When we assess, we need to consider that established models offer some help with assessment, but patients inform the models too. The symptoms and behaviour do not always fit the models. So, at the Wolfson we believe it is paramount to continue to be holistic in our assessment and thinking, and use the patient and their specific injury to enlighten us on the nature and consequences of the breakdown for them.

In summary then, SLT assessment is the investigation of the consequences of brain injury in terms of motor, linguistic and cognitive-communication problems, but additionally it needs to consider the consequences of these for the person and their family. We must also use assessment results to develop our theory of communication disability, particularly in relation to cognitive-communication disorder, and have a duty to share our learning and expertise with our colleagues.

Rationale

Assessment can serve a number of purposes for a number of people (for example therapist, patient, family, multidisciplinary team), but it is important for both therapist and patient that the rationale for why and what the therapist is assessing is explicit. Choice of assessment may not be guided solely by a therapist's clinical reasoning (for example, about neurology and expected difficulty) or observation, but by comments made by a patient's wife who has noticed that her husband does not pick up on the nuances of interaction and subtleties of language as he did prior to the onset of his aphasia. Traditionally, we would expect to complete a language assessment for someone presenting with aphasia. However, in this case use of The Awareness of Social Inference Test (TASIT) may be indicated and justified in addition.

Furthermore, not to assess must be based on rationale; it may not be appropriate to go through a battery of communication assessments with someone who has been admitted from an acute bed and only recently completed assessment, or someone who is coming into the unit for a short stay. In such cases it may be appropriate to focus on informal, indirect assessment and information gathering from other sources. Clear documentation of rationale is important for all cases.

Liaison and use of qualitative and quantitative assessments

Information gathering from previous SLT, the multidisciplinary team, relatives and nursing staff plays an important role as do questioning and exploring with the patients themselves. Parr *et al* (2001) discuss the qualitative interview and how it guides the therapists to the meaning of the disorder to the person. It offers the chance to explore whether assessments are a true reflection of communication behaviour in all situations. We must take the information we glean from traditional assessment and use it alongside the qualitative information we can obtain from a variety of sources in order to build a comprehensive and true picture of the communication disability that person experiences. This will help to ensure that the rehabilitation setting is a reflection of the real world, as far as possible. Within this process, key areas to explore are consistency, variety of needs, ability to express self with new people and getting needs met.

Baseline and outcome measures

The SLT department at the Wolfson has found it useful to establish a set of assessments from which we choose the most appropriate tools. This ensures a core, consistent and equitable approach for our patients and provides us with outcome measures that we can audit and use to analyse our service more closely. This approach follows the theory of assessment, therapy and reassessment to evaluate progress, but also considers qualitative information. We use a variety of assessment tools and patient-specific outcome measures to demonstrate treatment efficacy. Goal planning is integral to the patient's journey and a useful outcome measure. However, in order to ensure consistency and equity of input, minimum standards for pre and post therapy assessment have been devised, to be used in addition to goal planning. These are tailored to the individual according to the underlying impairment.

Outcome measures in the form of communication tables and scores are used to document outcomes of therapy from pre and post therapy assessment, in addition to goal attainment. The outcome measures in use by the SLT department aim to demonstrate the outcome of therapy at all levels, from impairment through to wellbeing, as outlined by Enderby *et al* (2006, see Table 1).

Table 1 Levels of therapy and example approaches

Level of therapy	Examples
'Improve/remediate'	Tackling the underlying communication impairment, eg cognitive-communication disorder, phonological, semantic, syntactic, pragmatic, motor, sensory disorders
'Extend functional activity relating to performance'	Communicating ideas, relating stories, use of total communication strategies/augmentative communication systems/aids
'Develop strategies to accommodate the personal social disadvantage of the deficit'	Educating others and modifying attitudes, providing strategies for patients and caregivers, attending social events, sustaining a work role, maximising independence in communication situations
'Support the patient and caregivers during the adjustment phase'	Identifying upset or concern, providing counselling, encouragement and support

Adapted from Enderby *et al*, 2006

It is important for the measurement to be meaningful, that is, not to be focused on ticking boxes but on generating information that, when looked at altogether, can give an idea about whether progress has occurred in different areas. A key requirement of the outcome measurement system is for it to be clinically applicable; it has proved possible to integrate this system into regular clinical practice for use with a variety of patients with differing therapeutic goals and diagnoses. Therefore clinical viability of such a system is indicated.

A recent study (McIntosh *et al*, in press) has found that outcome measures are needed to measure patients' perception of change and to measure functional change. Objective and subjective measures are therefore vitally important.

Aid to planning and prioritisation: use of skill mix

The process of assessment aids the Wolfson SLT department in prioritising and managing its caseload and staffing allocation. A systematic, equitable approach is used to identify and establish an individual's needs level in terms of input. This is discussed in more depth in Chapter 3 'Specific individualised treatment'.

Interrater reliability

Interrater reliability is very important regardless of the work setting. However, in the specialist and fairly newly recognised field where we work (that is, cognitive-communication disorder) it is particularly important that we strive for reliability within our department and approach. This relates to scoring and interpretation of assessment results, and to the terminology we are using to describe our patients' presentation. While we recognise its importance, we admit that this is an area where we find it difficult to ensure that reliability is achieved at best practice level. Carrying out research and developing the area of specialist neurorehabilitation can only serve to support interrater reliability.

Education, feedback to the patient and insight raising

Education forms a strand of its own and is therefore talked about in depth further on. However, it is important to stress that assessment should not be used for the therapist's knowledge alone. Feeding back a person's performance on assessment is not only good practice, but is also therapeutically very valuable. It can aid insight raising and the process of adjustment, it can help with motivating the individual, provide support in explaining the rationale for therapy, and help to adjust the expectations of the individual and their family and friends. Information gathered through assessment, both SLT and from the wider multidisciplinary team, can be used to open up or support discussions around the difficult subject of prognosis.

What we do

PRE-ADMISSION PHASE

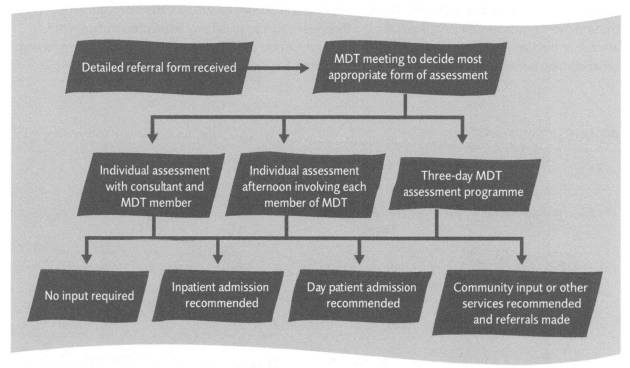

Figure 2 Assessment process at pre-admission phase

Assessment not only guides SLT work with patients admitted to the Wolfson, it also plays a part prior to their stay. Every patient comes to a pre-admission assessment with members of the multidisciplinary team to establish their needs and suitability for rehabilitation (see Figure 2). These assessments are different: what is needed is determined by the information received from the referrers, each of whom is asked to fill in a detailed referral form. The assessment format ranges from a one-hour individual joint assessment, involving two or three members of the multidisciplinary team, to a three-day assessment (the Wolfson Cognitive Assessment Programme) whereby a thorough multidisciplinary team assessment is carried out and goals are negotiated for an inpatient stay or a block of outpatient therapy, if considered appropriate. The assessment process can help to identify services and input that need to be offered before admission – for example, management of depression or referral for alcohol rehabilitation – to ensure the patient derives maximum benefit from their admission.

A unique function of the Wolfson assessment process is to identify the most appropriate service provision for that individual at that time. Some referrals are made with the intention of seeking advice and guidance from the multidisciplinary team, so the outcome of the pre-admission assessment may be provision of guidelines, recommendations and advice for the referrer. We are fortunate to be in a position where we can help move things forward for the patient on their journey, for example, by referring on for therapy in the community.

At assessment consideration is given to whether the intensive multidisciplinary programme is appropriate, whether there are goals to work towards or whether some other treatment or community-based input may be a more suitable option. Sometimes goals have been established prior to assessment with therapists who have been treating patients in the acute setting or the community. Similarly, the Wolfson may refer the patient on to the community team, as the goals identified may appear more achievable that way. The level of function, prognosis, referrer's motivation for referral and patient and family perspective all influence the outcome of the assessment.

Inclusion of SLT in the pre-admission decision making is important to support and advocate for those patients with specific communication difficulties, and also to influence the profile of patients attending the Wolfson. (It is common for patients with severe physical disability to be viewed as having rehabilitation needs but not perhaps those with primary linguistic or psychological needs.)

ADMISSION PHASE

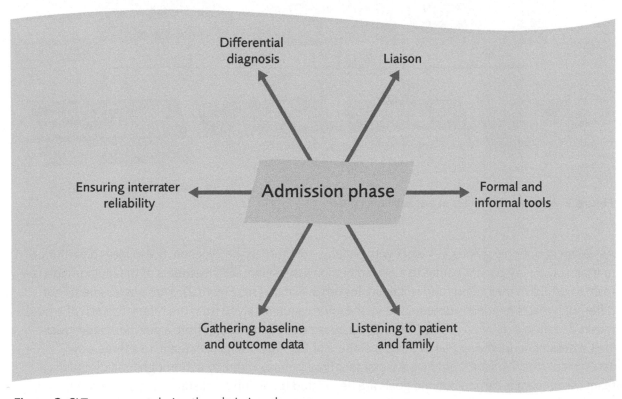

Figure 3 SLT assessment during the admission phase

Liaison

As we have stated, it is important to gather as much information as possible to aid therapy planning. We spend a significant amount of time allocated to a patient in 'indirect assessment work' (see Figure 3): for example, phone calls with previous therapists to explore prior assessment and input; discussion with family and friends to explore pre brain injury characteristics and communication; liaison with nursing and healthcare colleagues regarding eating and drinking; discussing performance in daily activities (for example, washing and dressing) and in assessments with our multidisciplinary team colleagues. This liaison work is valuable time spent to add to the communication and swallowing profile of the patient.

At the Wolfson we have developed a communication checklist we have found to be particularly useful with our low-level patients (see Appendix). This is an informal observation tool that can be completed by a range of people involved with the patient, from family through to nursing staff, and gathers information about areas such as basic interaction, levels of activity and stimulation, demonstration of preference and expressing basic needs.

Informal and formal: the importance of listening to the patient and family

We use a wide range of assessment tools and methods in a variety of situations, and aim to consider all quantitative and qualitative information that both formal and informal tools provide. We aim to be holistic with our choice of formal assessments and have available a wide range of published language and communication assessments (see Appendix).

We obtain a great deal of our assessment information from family and friends as well as from the patients themselves. In addition to completing and feeding back results of formal assessments, we make use of mind maps to build a picture of pre and post brain injury self and communication, and use informal rating scales that we have devised over time, or that are devised specifically for an individual (for example confidence rating, rating of loudness and intelligibility). Self-rating scales are valuable in assessing level of awareness and provide useful baselines for comparison and reassessment during and post therapy. Use of video (with and without rating scales) similarly provides essential assessment information as a baseline and outcome measure and to feed back to patient and family. We regularly make videos in various settings, for example of a group, at a mealtime, with a member of the family or an identified friend, in order to get a real-life picture of communication and/or swallowing skills, and in multidisciplinary team sessions. These are then used for ongoing assessment and as therapy tools, including for feedback purposes.

Questionnaires provide us with valuable information at various stages throughout the therapy process. We make use of published questionnaires, such as the MCLA family questionnaire and BICRO-39, in addition to patient-specific questionnaires we may have developed with the patient about a particular area of communication. Questionnaires may be disseminated to family members, friends and members of the team according to the information required.

A recent development at the Wolfson is the use of a structured process of assessment and reassessment with our conversation groups. We have been running groups as part of our service delivery for many years. We have always strongly believed them to be effective alongside individual sessions, but have had little evidence to prove this beyond anecdotal observations and client feedback. We developed a structure that would be more systematic and therefore easier to replicate and that would make it easier to demonstrate outcome through assessment and reassessment. We wanted an assessment tool that would reflect overall performance in conversation as well as the specific aspect defined by the client's goal (negotiated prior to or within the group). Previous therapists at the Wolfson had devised a 'communication wheel' to map a person's abilities. We decided to trial an adapted version as an observation schedule to be completed at the start and end of the group in order to demonstrate outcomes (see Figure 4 overleaf). This has proved a useful and systematic approach to measuring the qualitative information we observe.

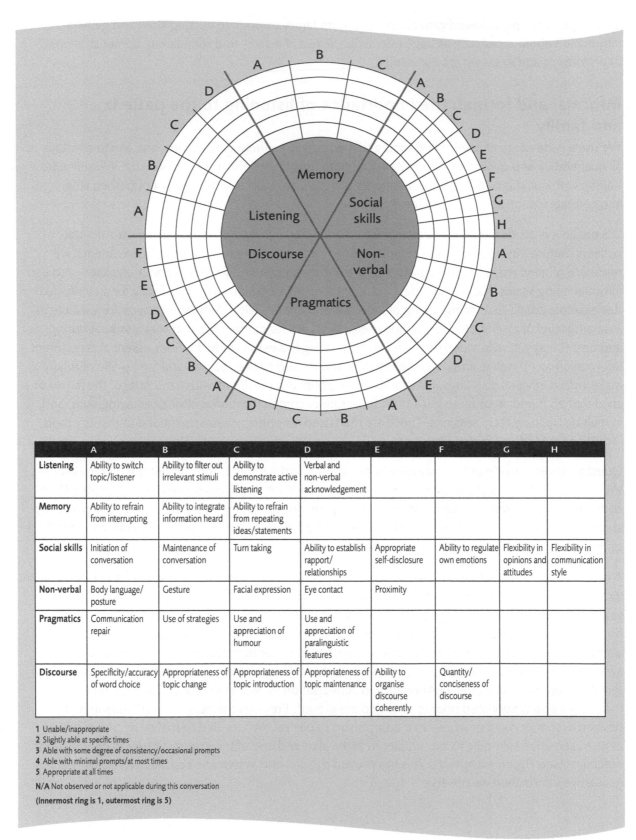

	A	B	C	D	E	F	G	H
Listening	Ability to switch topic/listener	Ability to filter out irrelevant stimuli	Ability to demonstrate active listening	Verbal and non-verbal acknowledgement				
Memory	Ability to refrain from interrupting	Ability to integrate information heard	Ability to refrain from repeating ideas/statements					
Social skills	Initiation of conversation	Maintenance of conversation	Turn taking	Ability to establish rapport/ relationships	Appropriate self-disclosure	Ability to regulate own emotions	Flexibility in opinions and attitudes	Flexibility in communication style
Non-verbal	Body language/ posture	Gesture	Facial expression	Eye contact	Proximity			
Pragmatics	Communication repair	Use of strategies	Use and appreciation of humour	Use and appreciation of paralinguistic features				
Discourse	Specificity/accuracy of word choice	Appropriateness of topic change	Appropriateness of topic introduction	Appropriateness of topic maintenance	Ability to organise discourse coherently	Quantity/ conciseness of discourse		

1 Unable/inappropriate
2 Slightly able at specific times
3 Able with some degree of consistency/occasional prompts
4 Able with minimal prompts/at most times
5 Appropriate at all times

N/A Not observed or not applicable during this conversation

(Innermost ring is 1, outermost ring is 5)

Figure 4 Conversation group wheel developed at the Wolfson

We are fortunate at the Wolfson to have access to computer facilities and specific language-based computer programs from which we can obtain additional information to support our diagnoses and hypotheses formulation. We make regular use of *StepByStep Words* (Steps Consulting, 2005) and *React2* (Mitchell *et al*, 2008), which provide useful ongoing reassessment information in addition to being therapy resources.

We consider all informal information and use it to guide us, taking note of evidence that comes up in real-life situations, such as how the individual communicates their needs to the nursing staff during their morning routine, or how the husband and wife communicate and deal with a situation that has come up at home. We find our observations during different communication environments are also useful assessment tools: for example, comparing performance in individual therapy sessions with that seen in a group where the demands are different. It is recognised within the department that trips 'out and about' during the admission provide useful qualitative information, so we regularly accompany people out into the community, to locations 'normal' to their life. This might be a simple trip to the local newsagent's, or breakfast in a 'greasy spoon' café, or a visit to an art gallery or favoured football club. To obtain the most relevant and meaningful observations, we must park our prejudices and be willing to participate in activities in keeping with the person's normal life experiences.

Differential diagnosis

A useful approach to aiding differential diagnosis is through the use of therapy groups. Participants in the groups often have a mix of difficulties rather than being disorder-specific (particularly our conversation and education groups), and observing these difficulties in a group situation can help us identify if a problem has a more linguistic or cognitive basis.

Outcome measures

The SLT department has been trialling an integrated outcome measurement system to capture change arising from a broadened intervention approach. 'Broadened' intervention can include working on identity or confidence, or aiming for awareness and self-actualisation through education. Therefore it is of particular importance to capture the patient's own perception of change in the system. By choosing a set of outcomes and itemising the parameters, it is possible to demonstrate the change that we know happens, both through our clinical assessment and because patients tell us so. Use of the self-report enables the patient's 'voice' to form part of the baseline and outcome ratings.

Interrater reliability

We acknowledge that this is an area of ongoing development and are very aware of the fact that, even with the scoring systems of published assessments, performance can be differently interpreted. To try to minimise the differences and raise reliability, we carry out joint sessions and provide second opinions as well as making time for departmental training and regular education sessions, for example, on phonetic transcription, watching patients' videos and carrying out group ratings with our conversation group wheels. Training students also helps to highlight the importance of this area and encourages us even more to make time for comparing our approach and interpretations.

Developing a screening tool

We have discussed the complexities of differential diagnosis and the increasing evidence in the literature relating to cognitive-communication disorder. Although speech and language therapists are starting to recognise and treat cognitive-communication disorder, information on what to assess and what treatment to provide is not as readily available or as well researched as that available for people with aphasia, dysarthria or apraxia. It is therefore important as a first step to identify the frequency of cognitive-communication disorder in order to later ensure equitable access to appropriate assessment and treatment services. As a specialist centre, we have a duty to share our knowledge with others. The SLT department is currently involved in a research project investigating the incidence of cognitive-communication disorder in stroke patients and relating this to site of lesion. From this, we are aiming for validation of a stroke screening tool to enable accurate identification of patients with cognitive-communication disorder.

Conclusions

It is important to recognise and remember that assessment is an ongoing and vital process throughout the period of rehabilitation. The process of therapy must be seen as part of assessment and vice versa, and not one that stops as soon as the formal assessment forms have been completed and scored. Furthermore, it should be seen as a holistic, patient-centred process that is transparent to the patient and their family as being part of the rehabilitation journey, regularly guiding and directing the therapy approaches as things change over time.

Case study: John

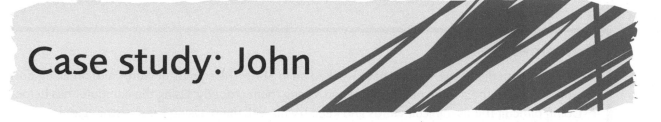

John's assessment and feedback strand

A man of 43 with aphasia, dyspraxia and cognitive-communication disorder following a stroke.

Pre-admission assessment phase

- John was assessed on 21 August 2007 by the clinical neuropsychologist and the speech and language therapist.
- He was accompanied by his wife and was asked a wide range of questions relevant to multidisciplinary rehabilitation.
- He presented with a left MCA infarct (Jan. 2007) secondary to carotid artery dissection and colloid cyst at the foramen of Munro.
- On assessment, he was found to have a right-sided weakness, aphasia, right homonymous hemianopia, hearing impairment, dyspraxia, cognitive impairment and executive functioning problems.
- Outcome of assessment was a recommendation that John be admitted for a period of inpatient neurorehabilitation of not more than 12 weeks.

Assessment on admission

- John was admitted on 8 October 2007. He was assessed formally and informally.
- Initial interview on day 1
- Client admission self-report: 'First thing in the morning I am fine, then later on my ability is worse. My real problem is saying words, but there is some difficulty thinking of the words. I can't say long sentences – it's not about remembering what thinking, it's trying to find the word. My understanding is pretty good. Genuinely quite good at thinking and listening to people. My people skills are still there.'
- Video baseline
- Comprehensive Aphasia Test (CAT)

Assessment feedback

- Reduced comprehension at high level, eg embedded sentences
- Word-finding difficulties evident in task and conversation
- Attempts to use strategies, eg writing the first letter
- Formal assessment: reduced verbal fluency, written and spoken comprehension reduced at complex sentence level, reading, repetition and naming severely impaired; evidence of conduite d'approche
- Feedback given via simplified cognitive neuropsychology model (Ellis & Young, 1998); video feedback deemed to be inappropriate due to John's emotional state

Outcomes

- Self-report on discharge, 'What I have worked on in SLT': 'The sounds of words and breaking down words to make them more remind them and saying them properly. Using the computer has helped. Doing difficult things, difficult words and keep trying with them. Using various strategies to get my speech correctly, make it more flow ... Education was very good and important.' Progress made: 'My speech has got better. More words together.'

- CAT on discharge: improved scores on single word naming and sentence comprehension

- Significant improvement in personalised rating scale (total score from 10.5 – 19.7); goal achieved to more than expected level

2 Goal planning

Goal planning is not a new concept, particularly in the field of rehabilitation; the literature refers to goal planning as far back as the 1970s. However, goal planning forms a very important and explicit strand of rehabilitation at the Wolfson. Without identifying goals with our patients we cannot truly establish priorities for therapy or indeed motivate our patients to continue with the undoubtedly challenging and often frustrating process of rehabilitation.

Goal planning is a flexible framework within which each patient's strengths, needs and wants can be assessed and managed. It enables each admission to be smoothly coordinated through interdisciplinary working. This involves partnership between the team of health professionals and the patient and family in a participatory, collaborative and coordinated approach in order to share decision making concerning the direction of rehabilitation and relevant health issues.

The process of goal planning aims to increase the patient's and family's involvement in their rehabilitation programme and reduce their dependency on the team and the 'institution'. It aims to be a transparent service, clear to all involved. In so doing, it ensures an effective and efficient admission for the patient and results in their seamless transition into the community.

Goal areas expressed by patients, and then discussed and negotiated with the multidisciplinary team, are unique and can be multifaceted: for example, clear/fuzzy, realistic/unrealistic, in need of revision, open to change over time/with more experience, easier/more difficulty to articulate. It is the role of the chairperson, the multidisciplinary team and the patient, with their family and friends, to communicate clearly with each other to make the goal-planning process work for that person. Part of this involves supporting the writing of goals that are not only meaningful to the patient, but also measurable.

Guiding principles

There are four key principles that form the basis of effective goal planning at the Wolfson.

1 Patient and family involvement

The patient and, just as importantly, their family and friends are central to the success of neurorehabilitation and therefore to the process of goal planning. Consequently, they need to be involved at all stages as much as possible. This includes being involved in the identification of strengths and problems, in the setting of goals, in appreciating what action needs to be taken to achieve these goals and in reviewing progress. This allows the individual, with their family and friends, to gain greater control over their own rehabilitation and increases their commitment to and engagement with the process. It also provides opportunities for developing their insight into the recovery and therapy processes and helps them prepare for discharge.

Goal planning provides opportunities for the patient, family, friends and the multidisciplinary team to develop more open lines of communication, a better appreciation of each other's perspectives and access to support and strategies to tackle issues jointly. It is important to note that patients will vary in the extent to which they will want to involve their family and friends, and this should be respected.

2 Identifying strengths and problems

In order to identify goals, the multidisciplinary team first needs to be aware of an individual's strengths and problems within the context of their own family, social and employment context, and their future aspirations. In addition, all possible resources available to the patient need to be identified.

At the pre-admission assessment the multidisciplinary team sets out to formulate an idea of an individual's strengths, needs and wants. These can change prior to admission and therefore need to be clarified when the person begins their rehabilitation. As soon as the patient arrives it is possible for the multidisciplinary team to assess these areas more thoroughly in collaboration with the individual and their family and friends. This gives everyone clearer information with which to plan the rehabilitation programme and to set goals.

3 Goal negotiation and writing

Goals must be patient-centred and the process of establishing the goals must be explicit for the patient, their family and friends and members of the team in order to ensure everyone involved is proceeding in the same direction. Negotiating goals is about producing a desired change in behaviour. It is important to remember that small changes (short-term goals) may be more easily achieved than big changes (long-term goals). This helps to avoid failure and may help to keep everyone motivated. It is the skill of the multidisciplinary team to help the patient translate their needs, wants and aspirations into clear goals.

Discussion of long-term goals provides a platform to begin the exploration of the patient's understanding of their injury and potential recovery, and their expectations. Issues relating to managing dependence may be highlighted in addition to the patient's support needs and network. It can help to facilitate discussion about role changes and disability, loss and the grief reaction, and thus facilitate the process of psychosocial adjustment. The process of negotiating goals can be both powerful and emotional for the patient and their family, as they begin the process of identifying the path forward and also the challenges they will encounter along the way.

It is acknowledged that goals of personal value enhance an individual's ability to engage in rehabilitation. Recent self-efficacy based approaches aim to put the individual in the 'driving seat' through personal 'real-life' goal identification. For example, 'Stepping out' (Jones, 2008), a stroke self-management programme which empowers individuals to take control of their daily lives, is based on the premise that self-efficacy interventions can influence quality of life (Robinson-Smith et al, 2000).

For a goal to be understandable by all involved and measurable, it should reflect who will be doing what, under what conditions, to what degree of success, within what period of time. Main goals are referred to as long-term (that is, to be achieved by discharge). A long-term goal reflects a change in participation and activity for the patient in their life and may include the broad domains of home, leisure, social, relationships, occupation/self-occupation, self-care, physical change and/or cognitive change. Short-term goals are the smaller steps, or steps to achievement, that lead towards the long-term goal. These may be focused at an impairment level.

4 Team working

A criterion for admission to the Wolfson is that an individual will require input from more than one discipline. The neurological injury sustained by an individual impacts on all areas of their life (social, occupation, activities of daily living, mobility, self-care, sexual function and psychological wellbeing). It would be unrealistic to expect one professional to have the expertise necessary to meet the individual needs in all of these areas; indeed, a critical factor is to create an environment of interdisciplinary care.

Such interdisciplinary working involves acknowledging the overlap between professional disciplines with a 'greater sharing of duties and responsibilities ...' (Department of Health, 2001). Successful teams may possess combinations of skills that no single individual demonstrates.

Collaboration in goal planning not only helps to ensure that there is carry-over from one area to another, but also avoids duplication. However, due to the number of people involved, a coordinated approach is crucial to ensure that the *whole* team is aware of the direction in which the individual is going at any point in time. Interdisciplinary working should be supported by clear and user-friendly documentation. Team members' roles and boundaries should be communicated regularly throughout admission up to the point of discharge, so that it is clear who is doing what, where and when.

What we do

Essential to the successful working of the multidisciplinary team at the Wolfson is the chairperson. In brief, they are responsible for coordinating the goal-planning process through both written and verbal communication, attending to the process as well as the tasks and ensuring that at all times the patient is at the centre of all activities throughout their stay. This is not to say the chairperson has sole responsibility for that patient. Through our chair training sessions we acknowledge the role of the chairperson, but perhaps more importantly, we highlight the roles and responsibilities of the others within the treating team (such as liaison, support, open communication, accepting responsibility and seeing actions through).

Currently we are working towards a 'goal attainment scaling' framework for our goal planning and writing. Goal attainment scaling (GAS) is a technique for evaluating individual progress towards goals. Despite recognition of GAS as a clinical outcome assessment technique in other clinical professions (Kiresuk *et al*, 1994), the current debate on measuring client progress and outcome measurement in communication disorders has largely ignored GAS (Schlosser, 2003). However, we have generally found it to be useful to date, especially where we work alongside our multidisciplinary team colleagues to ensure goals remain patient-specific and relevant.

When setting a GAS goal we are asking the patient to achieve a specific target over a three-month period or another agreed time span (for example, from admission to discharge). Goals should represent the most probable outcome for the agreed span of time, indicating what is most likely to happen, not what would be most desirable.

Although goal planning is a flexible framework, there are six key stages in the process, as shown in Figure 5 (overleaf).

1 Plan of assessment meeting

The plan of assessment will ensure that *everyone* knows what they will be assessing up to the first goal-planning meeting. It involves only the treating team and serves to provide the multidisciplinary team with a focus. The plan helps to avoid duplication of assessment and to ensure that the most appropriate people are carrying out those assessments. The meeting lasts between 15 and 30 minutes and is ideally carried out within the first week of admission.

2 First goal-planning meeting to establish goal areas

Within two weeks of admission the chairperson convenes a meeting with the patient, their family and/ or friends as appropriate and all relevant team members. It is important to remember that the number

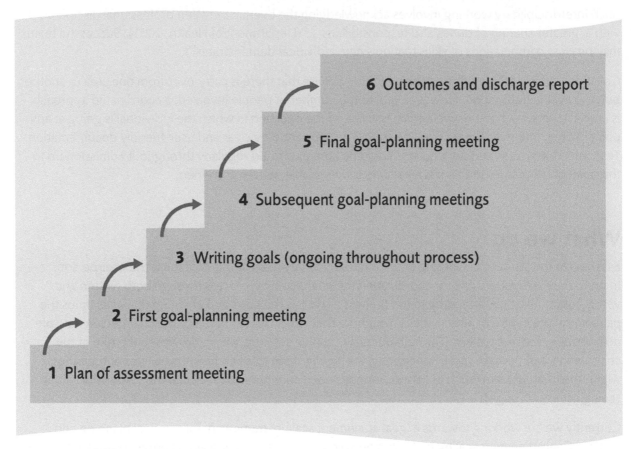

Figure 5 Six key stages of goal planning

of people can vary according to the patient's wants, needs and preferences. Also, the environment may vary according to the formality/informality/style with which the patient feels most comfortable.

The first task at this meeting is to complete a list of the patient's strengths and problems. The patient, together with the multidisciplinary team, can then start to identify areas in their life that they are keen to focus on while working at the Wolfson. In the first meeting it may not be possible to set any specific long-term goals, but if not, then goal areas should at least be discussed, which will then be formalised as GAS goals. One or more 'problems' from the problem list may correlate with specific goals, while others may require plans of action instead. Ideally, the multidisciplinary team will already, as individual disciplines, have had some discussion of goals with the patient in their own sessions prior to the meeting. It is crucial that this goal-planning meeting should hold no surprises for the patient.

The meeting will last for one hour and either the team can meet for the first half hour, with the patient joining for the second half hour, or the patient and family/friends can participate for the whole hour. This decision is at the discretion of the chairperson and the team in full discussion with the patient.

3 Writing goals

As discussed earlier, for a goal to be understandable by all involved and measurable, it should reflect who will be doing what, under what conditions, to what degree of success, within what period of time. It is important that the patient has ownership of their goals and we strongly advocate that each individual is given a written copy of their negotiated goals. These can then be referred to at any stage during the rehabilitation.

Examples of long-term goals

'John will return home alone with three daily visits from carers in the community in 10 weeks.'

'John will make 12–16 entries a week in his diary [as a memory aid] by discharge.'

'June will independently plan and attend a meal out with her sister once a week by discharge.'

'On a daily basis John will walk 10 metres inside and outside with a stick by discharge.'

'Gill will discuss school, soaps and friends with her daughter once a day by discharge.'

'Joe will eat a chopped/mashed consistency Christmas dinner with his family by discharge.'

'By discharge Malcolm will use a range of "total communication" strategies, particularly his communication file, in order to participate in a social activity of his choice.'

Examples of short-term goals or 'steps to achievement'

'Susan will correct her posture four times in a five-minute period using a mirror in Physiotherapy.'

'June will use the Yellow Pages to identify two restaurants to contact within two weeks.'

'John will make a summary in a diary at the end of each therapy session with verbal prompts during the next two weeks.'

4 Subsequent goal-planning meetings

All long-term goals and steps to achievement are reviewed at fortnightly team meetings involving the patient and relevant family and/or friends who have been identified early on in the goal-planning process. To direct the patient through their journey, short-term goals or steps to achievement for the proceeding two weeks are set at this meeting.

We find it useful to think about inreach and outreach during the latter stages of the goal-planning process. For those patients who will be referred on for further rehabilitation in the community or for continuing care, it can be helpful to invite the relevant professionals to attend the goal-planning meetings. Not only does this help to ensure smooth transition and carry-over of goals, it also allows the patient and their family to 'put a face to a name' for what is often a daunting next stage.

5 Final goal-planning meeting

At the final team meeting long-term goals will be reviewed. This will allow everyone to ensure that all identified areas of need have been dealt with. It provides the multidisciplinary team, the patient and their family and friends with a useful opportunity for 'endings' and to identify possible future goal areas, for example, those that can be included in the referral to community teams and in handover to carers. Again, we encourage the involvement of community teams and care agencies at this stage.

6 Discharge report including outcomes

Experience has taught us that beginning the report writing early in the rehabilitation process is beneficial. Multidisciplinary reports are multifaceted and often lengthy documents that we set out to complete by discharge. It is not the sole responsibility of the chairperson to complete the report; each member of the multidisciplinary team has equal responsibility to achieve this deadline. However, it is the role of the chairperson to coordinate and ensure the report is well written and completed in a timely manner.

Conclusions

Setting goals or personal targets is a key part of many people's lives, ranging from smaller goals such as going to post a letter or shopping, to more ambitious life goals such as completing a college course or retiring to another country. However, people vary in the extent to which they are 'goal-focused'. Every patient, family member and friend will have a different perspective on what 'goal planning' means when they come to the rehabilitation centre. The multidisciplinary team needs to take these factors into consideration when working with the individual and their family and friends. It is by establishing goals of personal value to the client that Malec (1999) believes we are more likely to securely engage them in the rehabilitation process.

Goal planning is a simple process that takes a high level of skill and time to negotiate and work with usefully. It should not be seen as a predetermined series of steps or tasks, but a framework within which an individual can be guided forwards towards their future.

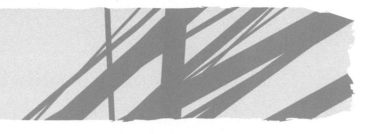

Case studies

John's goal-planning strand

- Started goal negotiation on 23 October 2007, continued until 2 November: 'I would like to get my words so good I will be able to have a normal conversation.'

- 'To evaluate myself on my communication rating scale and score 15–18 points out of 25.' Rating scale included items about speed and accuracy of word finding and involvement in family decision making.

- 'To have established a role at home.'

- 'To be able to clearly explain about my stroke and subsequent difficulties.'

- 'To have identified at least four activities I can participate in on discharge.'

Susie's goal-planning strand

A woman of 71 with receptive and expressive aphasia and cognitive-communication disorder following two strokes.

- Started goal negotiation on 10 May 2009 and continued over a number of weeks: 'I want to talk and get it right and do my life again.'

- 'During a conversation with the speech and language therapist about my family and friends, I will get their names right most of the time' (measured as 65–70% accuracy).

- 'I will order my choice of food and drink when out for lunch, using whatever strategies I need to communicate.'

- 'To be able to find three items I want in a supermarket (from a shopping list).'

- 'To do my housework (washing, hanging out and ironing) with supervision only.'

- 'To be able to make a familiar meal independently.'

- 'To complete a cognitive assessment and understand my strengths and weaknesses.'

- 'I will ask the nurses for my medications at the correct time of day.'

3 Specific individualised treatment

Tailoring the rehabilitation process to fit the individual patient is a key element of our philosophy. The individualised treatment approach places the patient at the centre of their rehabilitation. This allows the rehabilitation plan to reflect and recognise the patient's personal aims and motivations and in doing so improves engagement of the individual in the rehabilitation process. A specific individualised treatment plan is made up of 'core' elements – treatments provided to all patients – and 'available' elements – treatments that may be useful for individual patients. The plan is governed by a set of guiding principles that influence our decision making at all stages of rehabilitation.

Guiding principles

Prognosis

Working with relevant literature, medical diagnoses and SLT diagnoses in mind, we generate a concept about prognosis for each individual. While this acts as a guide for rehabilitation, we do not allow it to restrict, particularly when viewing the future, as communication impairment is a long-term disability and a period of rehabilitation presents only a snapshot of function.

We believe transparency is important in addressing prognosis, and providing the patient with this information enables them to better understand their disability and participate in rehabilitation. Planning of therapy is done with long-term prognosis in mind: for example, considering if therapy may be more relevant to the individual in the context of their home and thus an early referral to community services is indicated. Prognosis and outcome are viewed as separate and we endeavour not to be straightjacketed by prognosis. Owing to the status of the Wolfson, we have the opportunity to work with patients who are perceived as having a poor prognosis. We believe it is possible to say it is never 'too late' to attempt rehabilitation. For example, if a patient has had some impairment-based therapy, but no education or strategy facilitation, there are clear goals to change outcome, regardless of prognosis.

Use of interpreters

Understanding the impact of a patient's previous level of English is highly relevant to the rehabilitation process, and liaising with family members and friends may be important not only in investigating this but also in offering support around interpretation. We view the need for interpreters not as a barrier or prevention to rehabilitation but as an area to work around and with. We acknowledge the reality of the difficulty of using trained interpreters and for this reason we make use of family members and staff. Furthermore, it is preferable to use family members as they will be conversing with the patient regularly.

International classification framework

The International Classification of Functioning, Disability and Health (ICF; World Health Organization, 2002) aims to provide a unified and standard language and framework for the description of health and health-related states (see Figure 6 overleaf). These domains are described from the perspectives of the body, the individual and society in two basic categories: (1) body functions and structures, (2) activities and participation.

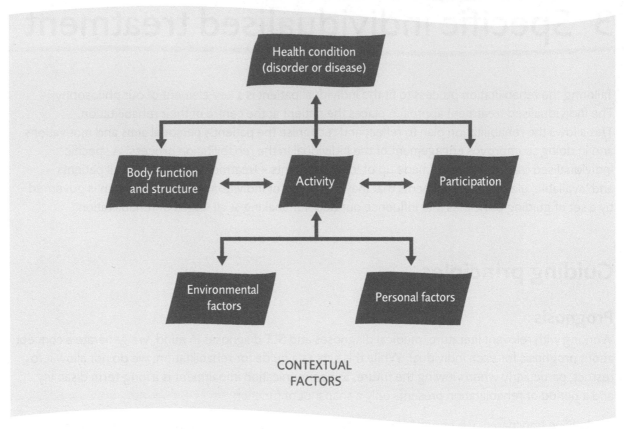

Figure 6 ICF classification. Adapted from World Health Organization, 2002

The ICF guides and informs our therapy; it is important for us to consider which level of the framework we are working at and to ensure that we have considered all levels. We consider this in conjunction with what is relevant to the individual at that time and what we recommend should be covered later, independently or in a different setting.

Individual clinician's judgement but with a shared team input

We have an eclectic approach to decision making within SLT and encourage frequent open forums in which we can debate issues and consider differing opinions. Decisions such as increasing an individual patient's session time are made as a team; this avoids decisions being overly influenced by the treating therapist, who may have an individual bias. There are opportunities for frequent joint working to provide support and share ideas.

Patient-centred working

Patient-centred working is achieved through joint goal negotiation and by involving the patient in all aspects of decision making. By finding out about their life and what is important to them, we as clinicians are better able to make the patient's thoughts and feelings the number one priority. During rehabilitation the family is viewed as important, but the patient's needs are paramount and therefore we attempt to advocate for the patient. Ongoing monitoring of motivation and goals through the goal-planning process, continually checking that the patient is happy with therapy and providing them with space to bring up issues, help us to consider whether we are achieving a patient-centred rehabilitation journey.

Consent and readiness

All patients are encouraged to give consent for use of video, for family members to be contacted etc. We attempt to ensure that the individual understands the rationale behind therapy and is ready to participate. If the patient is not yet ready it may be appropriate to encourage progress towards readiness through insight building, family feedback or motivational interviewing.

Access to service and equity

All patients should have access to the SLT service if appropriate. Patients can be referred by anyone within the Wolfson – staff or family members – and we are able to screen patients when requested before embarking on the therapeutic process. In order to effectively manage the caseload, a prioritisation and needs level system can be used to support this process. This should be a flexible but directive guide and requires the caseload to be reviewed on a regular basis to ensure changing needs are acknowledged and met.

Interdisciplinary working

Orchard *et al* (2005) emphasise the importance of an interdisciplinary approach that is participatory, collaborative and coordinated when sharing decision making about health issues. Furthermore, they advocate a partnership between the team of health professionals and the client.

At the Wolfson, we strongly believe in this approach, but for ease we tend to use the term 'multidisciplinary team'. Within SLT we have recognised there are what we refer to as the 12 Cs of team working, which, when borne in mind, maximise the rehabilitation journey for the individuals involved.

Table 2 The 12 Cs of team working

1	Clear expectations	Role – of each team member and of the patient and their family/ friends
		Goals – making these explicit early on to direct the rehabilitation and aid the setting of expectations
		Diagnosis and prognosis – being guided by the neurological and communication diagnosis and making this explicit to all involved
		Service – '... people and their carers need information on the services and support available so they can take part in setting and meeting rehabilitation goals and manage the impact of their condition on their lives.' (Department of Health, 2005)
2	Clarity	Of team members' thinking
		Of our presentation of therapy and approaches
3	Context	Do members know why they are in the team?
4	Commitment	Are all team members taking responsibility?
5	Competence	Do team members feel they have got the right people in the team?
		Acknowledging where and who to turn to when a team member feels out of their depth; seeking additional advice and expertise

6	Charter	Vision and mission statement – and making this clear to all the team
7	Control	Does the team have sufficient freedom and empowerment to accomplish its charter?
8	Collaboration	Ensuring the team understand the group process, roles and responsibilities Goal negotiation involves the client, family and treating team
9	Communication	Clear lines of communication for all, which are assertive and involve negotiation Allocating a chairperson to coordinate and facilitate lines of communication Clear documentation of agreed actions
10	Creativity/ innovation	Thinking outside the box and being prepared to embrace novel, appropriate ideas
11	Conflict management	Recognising and acknowledging the conflict Finding help and support to manage it
12	Complementary skills	Recognising and being explicit about overlap of roles Ongoing education and discussion of roles and knowledge base

Real life: is it reflected in rehabilitation?

When formulating therapy plans it is essential to consider what is 'real life' for that patient. To ensure the therapy is meaningful and therefore motivating it must have relevance to the lives of the patients, their families and friends. Exploration of daily routines and tasks that the patient undertook at home, for leisure, socially and at work prior to the brain injury is a useful starting point. Ylvisaker & Feeney (2000a) discuss the importance of making the aim 'success in life' and advocate addressing activity and participation in order for new strategies and behaviour to become internalised.

Pathway

There may be occasions when our active involvement is not the most appropriate approach at that particular time along the patient's journey. We have found this more recently with the onset of short-term admissions to the Wolfson. Normally this pathway is for those individuals with chronic neurodisability, for example multiple sclerosis, who have been identified as likely to benefit from a short, intensive burst of rehabilitation. It is important that we spend time exploring the background before we go in 'with all guns blazing'. Someone with a chronic condition may already be under the care of a community speech and language therapist who has their communication and swallowing needs well managed, and for us to go in and start the whole process may be counterproductive and a waste of time for all involved. In such situations, inreach and outreach are vital; obtaining relevant information from relevant parties prior to admission will be of all-round benefit.

What we do: core and available approaches

There are a number of core elements of treatment that we apply to all patients who are accepted on the SLT caseload. Following on from the principles described above, this directs our way of working to ensure equal and fair access to services. We outline these core elements below, and they are followed by specific therapeutic approaches that are chosen according to patient need. This is not an exhaustive list of therapy, and it is certainly not the remit of this book to be a therapy manual, but we hope the examples we give will serve to illustrate our comprehensive and eclectic approach to specific individualised treatment.

CORE ELEMENTS OF TREATMENT

Needs levels and equality

We have a system of managing our SLT caseload that ensures it is equitable; this system is fundamental to therapy planning. Needs levels are allocated at a weekly update meeting and are based on BSRM guidelines (Royal College of Physicians & British Society of Rehabilitation Medicine, 2003) and guided by comparison with other tertiary rehabilitation units in order to benchmark services. This system also meets with criteria set in the *National Service Framework for Long-term Conditions* (Department of Health, 2005). Efficacy of therapy has long been debated and there is now convincing evidence that treatment is effective (Basso, 2005). Furthermore, studies such as that by Bhogal *et al* (2003) clearly show that the number and the intensity of therapy sessions are important factors in recovery, and that positive change is more likely to occur with greater amounts of therapy (Basso, 2005).

At the Wolfson, a high, medium or low clinical need is assigned to each person depending on a number of factors:

- severity of impairment
- level of disability and handicap
- time post onset
- motivation
- insight
- psychosocial factors
- potential for change
- therapy versus consultative model.

Needs levels are flexible and may change at various points during the course of admission, hence the need for a weekly review of the caseload.

Recent data from comparable centres suggest the ideal weekly SLT provision: high need – five hours per week; medium need – three hours per week; low need – two hours per week. Recent rehabilitation performance standards and quality markers established in the Department of Health's (2007) stroke strategy for high-quality, specialist inpatient rehabilitation set the standard as five 45-minute face-to-face sessions per week of SLT (in addition to occupational therapy and physiotherapy). This, we can assume, refers to provision for those patients with high clinical need. A Cochrane review (Turner-Stokes *et al*, 2009) of 16 studies found that, as a whole, patients with moderate to severe brain injury who received more intensive rehabilitation had earlier improvements. Of course, our service, like all services, has to respond to changes in caseload composition, staffing and departmental priorities and needs. While we strive to achieve this gold standard, we have to be flexible and adapt provision accordingly.

Assessment and outcome measures

As a minimum standard, on admission all patients complete outcome measures consisting of video baseline, client self-report, family questionnaire and appropriate formal assessment. Based on this information the patient is rated on a minimum of two parameters, for example comprehension and cognition. Additional formal or informal assessments are completed as required by the treating therapist or multidisciplinary team. Speech and language therapists also provide support during assessment in other disciplines, for example psychology. Flexibility within the assessment process is part of the individualised approach; informal assessment may be used with low-level clients. Assessment results are shared with patients and their families often to raise insight and inform goal planning and negotiation. Assessment results are also shared within the multidisciplinary team. These same measures are then repeated prior to discharge to provide the basis of outcomes and to inform the therapist and patient on progress, in addition to goal achievement.

Goal-directed treatment

Working towards person-centred specific goals ensures that therapy is measurable and progress or achievement can be clearly documented. Goals are negotiated with the patient to ensure they are relevant; this process promotes patient motivation and empowerment. Occasionally, it may be necessary to use non-negotiated goals, but these are often seen as an initial step towards independent goal setting. For example, an initial goal may be to raise insight, and after achieving this the patient may be better able to participate in negotiating further goals. The speech and language therapist has a specific role within the goal-planning process to help patients identify and express goals in the wider multidisciplinary team and at goal-planning meetings. All patients are allocated a chairperson to aid navigation through the goal-planning process. For patients with significant communication impairments a speech and language therapist chairperson may be allocated.

Individual and group therapy

All patients participate in a period of individual therapy initially for screening and/or assessment and goal negotiation. This may be carried out at the Wolfson, with additional assessment sessions in the community. Ongoing therapy is individual and/or group-based, and a variety of individual therapy approaches are used. Therapy always aims to work towards a specific goal.

Working with friends and family

It is not always possible to work with friends and family, and occasionally the client will not wish them to be included. Whenever appropriate, friends and family are involved at all stages of rehabilitation at the Wolfson. They will be encouraged to attend therapy sessions and may be invited to sessions without the patient. Friends and family are encouraged to view the Centre as a stepping stone to the future; this view may be supported by providing books and information, and answering questions. Encouraging links to the 'outside world' and helping friends and family look to the future may be achieved by referral on to community therapy and other services, assisting the family to explore local or national support groups, and coordinating 'out and about' sessions such as visits to restaurants or shopping centres.

Patient informed whenever possible

Working closely with the patient, it is important to explain the rationale for therapy and rehabilitation and to promote their understanding of the 'steps to achievement'.

Joint working and goals

Joint working is carried out within the SLT department, allowing therapists to develop their skills and gain a second opinion on specific issues. There may be situations where a therapy intervention would benefit from another therapist, for example, as a third person in conversation practice, to be a new person to give feedback, or to measure a specific parameter being worked on. Joint sessions within the multidisciplinary team include work with medics, with psychology, occupational therapy and physiotherapy departments, and with social work and nursing staff. Specific examples of joint working are supporting communication in discussions around consent to medical procedures, advising and supporting psychological assessment, breath support exercises with physiotherapy, the mealtime support group, and feeding with healthcare assistants. Often it will be useful to set joint goals in which steps to achievement may include joint or individual therapy and allocation of different tasks among the goal setters. Despite the importance placed on joint working, we also recognise the boundaries of our role as speech and language therapists. The most effective teams consist of a cohesive group of professionals who have different but complementary skills, and who trust and respect the expertise of other team members.

Speech and language therapists feel there is an important distinction between therapy and care, and therefore deem it respectful of the patient's dignity to take a step back from personal care.

Video

All patients are videoed (as long as consent is obtained) on admission and discharge as part of our outcome measurement system. A systematic video interaction evaluation tool is currently being developed to ensure interrater reliability and to provide us with a more robust outcome measure. Video is an invaluable tool, performing a multitude of functions within the rehabilitation process. It is frequently used to raise insight and promote change. It is also utilised in helping patients to develop a sense of identity, build confidence, receive direct feedback and be able to monitor their own progress, and to encourage them in self-advocacy. In a wider sense, video is also used to train conversation partners and raise the insight of friends and family, to hand over to carers, for teaching (for example, to demonstrate different communication diagnoses) and to provide specific treatment programmes (for example, developing comprehension of non-verbal communication by watching soaps). As a therapeutic tool video is so crucial that it should be used routinely in all rehabilitation services as a dynamic part of service delivery, in flexible and innovative ways.

AVAILABLE THERAPEUTIC APPROACHES

Available treatments may or may not be applied to individual patients, dependent on their goals and needs.

Therapy software

Within the department we have access to a number of computer-based impairment therapy packages, for example *StepByStep Words* (Steps Consulting, 2005), *Speech Sounds on Cue* (Bishop, 2004) and *React2* (Mitchell *et al*, 2008). As well as using them in our therapy sessions, we provide opportunities to work and progress through these programs independently or with a volunteer. Patients are able to access their own feedback and develop personal motivation and independence. In addition, clients may have computer-based goals such as accessing the internet or word processing, which often can be achieved through joint working with the occupational therapy department. We see a huge potential to use and develop the use of computers within the Wolfson, not only therapeutically but also to improve the range of leisure facilities. Offering computer games or facilities for emailing and researching on the internet can promote a return to activities the patient may have previously enjoyed. Recommending programs and facilitating access to internet-based support groups can help the patient to look to the future and manage their continued improvement after discharge. Steps Consulting (2005) highlights that such software enables delivery of more repetitive impairment-based word retrieval therapy tailored to the individual, releasing the therapist to focus on other aspects of communication.

Project work

Ylvisaker & Feeney (2000b) discuss the benefits of project work when working with individuals who lack motivation for therapy, particularly after traumatic brain injury (TBI). When lack of motivation is an issue and takes the form, 'I don't need to work on that; I can do it already', they suggest using an 'expert patient' approach and engaging the individual in working alongside the therapist to develop a manual or tip sheet or DVD designed to help others with similar difficulties. The goals of the project are to give the poorly motivated patient an expert role that enhances their motivation and creates opportunities for the student to practise the target skill while working on the project.

We have had success through use of such project work in supporting self-identity (Ylvisaker & Feeney, 2000b), engendering a sense of purpose and building roles. Individuals' pre-injury experience or skills can be utilised in tasks such as producing and giving presentations on the experience of brain injury and in rehabilitation and work-based activities such as researching and developing a resource of relevant information and lists of support agencies.

Independent work

The benefits of independent work can include improvements in self-motivation and the development of self-identity and confidence for the patient. It is also an effective method of managing time within the Wolfson, freeing up therapists' time and allowing the patient to make use of spare time they may have within their programme. Independent work may take the form of impairment-based assignments, computer use or projects as described above.

Independent working often targets integration into the community or a return to employment by encouraging the patient to practise tasks and providing a forum for feedback. Structuring of independent work programmes will include regular monitoring and reviews, and ensuring patients are aware of how to access support between reviews.

Outreach

An aim of the department is to work more closely with community teams. Currently, liaison with community teams is highly valued and community therapists often attend final goal-planning meetings. We recognise the value of being able to finish a job that is started and improving the 'smoothness' of the pathway through services. Outreach work may include negotiating future goals with patients and our community colleagues, assisting with return to work, developing links with other agencies, and informing new carers such as day centres and care homes.

Groups

Most patients access group therapy at some point during their admission. We have found that groups are useful in allowing peer feedback combined with therapist feedback, an opportunity for interaction, building friendships and sharing experiences. Referral to specific SLT groups is dependent on needs and goals, and the range of groups run at any one time is directed by needs within the caseload. Groups we run include the Brain Injury Education Group, Conversation Group, Total Communication, Social Group, Face Group (run jointly with the physiotherapy department), Mealtime Support Group, Lost for Words, Assertiveness Skills and Out and About. Groups are run by two therapists or a therapist and an assistant, and material for group sessions is available in 'group packs', reducing the need or time required for planning. However, groups are continually modified to accommodate patients' individual needs. We regularly evaluate the groups using informal evaluation forms and audit (James & Charles, 2008).

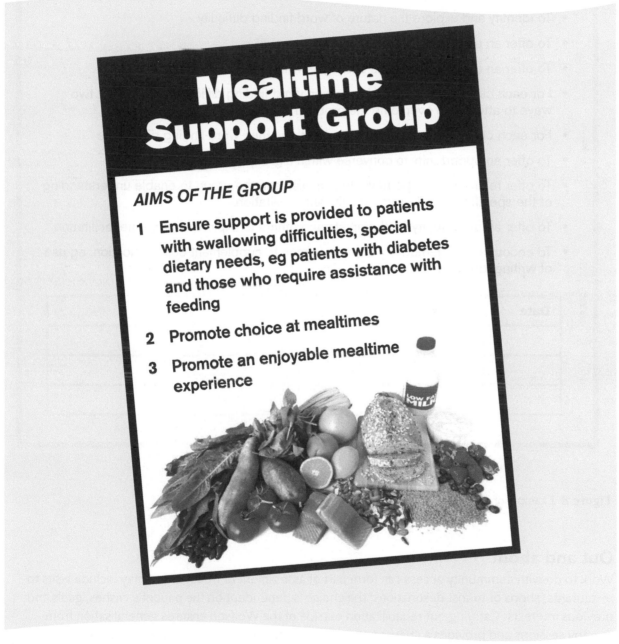

Figure 7 Example of a group poster

Lost for Words Group
Speech and Language Therapy

Aims

- To promote an understanding of specific word-finding difficulties

- To identify and explore the nature of word-finding difficulty

- To offer an opportunity to practise word retrieval

- To offer an opportunity to use strategies when stuck for a word

- For each client to be aware of their own word-finding difficulty and at least two ways to attempt to overcome the problem

- For each client to be able to explain to others their word-finding difficulties

- To offer an opportunity to converse within a group setting

- To offer relatives an opportunity to join clients in the group to enable understanding of the specific word-finding difficulty and facilitation

- To offer an opportunity for therapists and others to explore appropriate facilitation

- To encourage multi-modality communication to supplement communication, eg use of writing, drawing

Date	Topics

Figure 8 Example of a group documentation form

Out and about

Work to do with community access can form part of assessment or treatment. It may include visits to restaurants, shops or tourist destinations; the choice is dependent on the patient's wishes, goals and previous interests. Carrying out rehabilitation outside of the Wolfson ensures generalisation from therapy sessions and provides a chance to practise skills and increase the range of experiences. 'Out and abouts' are often important in aiding adjustment to the realities patients and their families will face on leaving the Centre. Sessions may be led by the speech and language therapist or involve the multidisciplinary team and may be conducted in a group or individually. Family members and friends may also be involved in the planning and/or the outing.

Counselling skills

Acknowledging the impact of neurological change on the patient and their family is an important part of SLT sessions. Observing and being open to recognising potential changes in mood, coping and emotional state is important to our intervention, particularly as SLT may offer an environment in which the patient feels able to open up about their thoughts and feelings. Referral to clinical psychology or to our counselling-trained speech and language therapist would support such a patient.

Day patient attendance

The current structure of the Wolfson allows for day patient attendance for higher-level patients who present with cognitive impairment. There are limited places available at any one time. The combination of multidisciplinary team inputs the patient receives will depend on their need. Within SLT, we typically offer a therapy group once a week to target a specific goal (for example, the conversation group). On occasion we may provide specific one-to-one therapy. Additionally, we are involved in the Wolfson's Cognitive Group Programme, a multidisciplinary programme of daily group sessions over a 12-week period. This is for patients who mostly acquired their brain injury some time before and who are living in the community, but not achieving their full potential.

Alternative and augmentative communication (AAC)

We have a role in assisting patients to access specialist communication aids and services and engage in trials of equipment. Advocating for patients where necessary and supporting them to make decisions regarding AAC is often vital to ensure that their potential to acquire and use a communication aid is maximised. Securing funding for communication aids is frequently difficult and may be a long process; at the Wolfson we liaise with community-based therapists to start the process as soon as possible. Where relevant we seek advice from specialist services such as the Charing Cross Assistive Communication Service (see Appendix for details). Currently, we use low tech communication aids more frequently than high tech. This is appropriate to the stage of rehabilitation reached by patients attending the Wolfson. Speech and language therapists may also work in conjunction with occupational therapists regarding the installation of environmental control systems. Knowledge of what is available and the referral processes involved is important.

Timeline process

Patients work with therapists and particularly with the SLT assistant to develop a visual timeline. This can be tailored to suit the individual's communication needs. The process forms part of insight building as patients can reflect on their life before impairment compared with now. Patients often benefit from the opportunity to 'tell their story', which can become a counselling tool. Used alongside psychology and with family members, the timeline can be developed as a strategy for patients with memory difficulties. The finished timeline can be used as a communication aid. Similar use of timelines in therapy can be found in the research of Parr et al (1997, 2001).

Training conversation partners

Training and education for the patient's family, although helpful, may not be sufficient to provoke change in communication behaviour. It is important to carry out specific tasks with specific conversation partners. Partners often require a great deal of encouragement to get involved and repeated practice is frequently necessary. Often therapy approaches may seem alien when applied to conversation with someone the partner has known and conversed with for years. Depending on the patient's social circle it may be relevant to work with members of the wider family, friends, children and colleagues. Video is a useful tool for raising insight, and developing rules and guidelines helps to provide structure and clarity to recommendations. Use of more structured approaches such as SPPARC (Lock *et al*, 2008) has also proved beneficial.

Case studies

John's specific individualised treatment strand

- Using *StepByStep Words* computer program with SLT volunteer (before goal negotiation)
- Conversation Group (James & Charles, 2008)
- Independent written tasks and worksheets
- Traditional impairment word-finding tasks
- Training in strategies for conversations
- Practising in-depth conversation, eg debate and discussion
- Telephone practice – role play taking messages
- Role play stressful situations, eg in the bank
- Community trip

Amelia's specific individualised treatment strand

A woman of 65 with severe verbal dyspraxia and global aphasia following a stroke.

- Using *StepByStep Words* and *Speech Sounds on Cue* computer programs with SLT volunteers
- Total Communication Group
- Traditional impairment therapy targeting single word comprehension and verbal output
- Sessions with SLT assistant working on reciting prayers, singing hymns
- Joint sessions with physiotherapy – standing to sing (goal of returning to church)
- Creating photo resource to aid conversation
- Training family in conversation strategies

4 Education

Educating an individual and those around them about their brain injury and communication disability is essential if we are to support them in engaging in the rehabilitation process. Perhaps more important is the role of education in the process of understanding, adjusting to and accepting the changes that have occurred. Spending time on information provision may seem to some to be a sacrifice of valuable 'traditional therapy' time. However, we see it as one of the core foundations of what we do.

Guiding principles

Provision of information

Within the field of counselling it is widely acknowledged that we need to hear news three to four times before we really begin to hear and assimilate that information and its meaning. It is not enough to assume that a patient and their family will have been given information about their brain injury at the acute phase and that this is sufficient information. Hoffman *et al* (2004) found that only 12–22 per cent of patients reported receiving written information about stroke before leaving hospital. What may seem like the basic details or repetition of information to us may be the dawning of new light and knowledge for a patient, and so the power of information should not be ignored.

Patient education materials (referred to as PEMs in the literature) provided in a written format have been found to have many benefits. According to Bernier (1993), they serve to supplement and reinforce verbal information; they offer message consistency; they can be referred to as and when the need arises and can be an effective method to support recall of information.

Furthermore, knowledge and understanding of brain injury and communication disability is a core foundation of empowerment. It enables patients to self-advocate, take control and assert themselves, thus raising self-esteem and confidence.

Personalised education

Ensuring that the information and education we provide meets the needs of the individual is key. A 'one size fits all' approach does not work when we are discussing the details of communication disability; while at an impairment level we can make comparisons between individuals, at an activity and participation level we cannot. How each person and their family and friends are affected is a unique experience. As Worrall *et al* (2005) concluded, people with aphasia have different information needs at various stages following the onset of their aphasia. This is, of course, true of any communication disability, and we must be mindful not only of level of impairment, but also of many factors, such as the patient journey, support, adjustment and pre-existing characteristics, when we personalise the education we provide.

Honesty is the best policy

We hold a strong belief that with all our patients honesty and openness about the neurological and communication diagnosis are essential and use of terminology should be adopted from the outset. Some patients, especially but not solely those with cognitive impairment, may be unaware of their condition and its cause; others may have heard the information but not fully taken it on board; while others may be in denial about their difficulties. Being honest and not covering up or colluding with an individual's misbelief aids a better understanding of a realistic prognosis, appropriate goal negotiation and, importantly, helps to facilitate the process of adjustment.

Education and goal negotiation

As we have stated elsewhere, person-centred education about brain injury and its consequences, particularly in relation to communication disability, should form a foundation layer of input if we are to successfully support the patient and their family in living with their communication disability. The importance of realistic goals has also been discussed. However, we are guided by the principle that without adequate knowledge and understanding of their own difficulties and the cause, an individual cannot truly engage in the goal-planning process. Raising a patient's awareness and insight into their own difficulties through ongoing education makes it easier to target areas of difficulty and therefore facilitate more effective ownership and involvement in the rehabilitation process.

Constructive feedback

While we strive for honesty, we are also very mindful of the emotional and psychosocial effects that hearing such information can bring. Feedback within an educational framework 'can inform individuals about the accuracy and progress of their performance. In addition, feedback can motivate patients by affecting their perception of competence and accomplishment' (Gauggel & Hoop, 2003, p442). We incorporate honest feedback into individual and group therapy and see it as an integral part of therapy. However, the timing of this information and how we provide it must be considered. The use of supportive counselling skills are essential as are opportunities to explore reactions to information and feedback, for example through further exploration, referral to psychology, sessions with family.

Family and friends

It perhaps goes without saying that family and friends are encouraged to be involved wherever possible. Education about brain injury leads to increased understanding and insight for all involved, thus providing the relevant tools often necessary to best support and encourage their relative who has been affected.

Knowledge and understanding about the impact of brain injury enable family and friends to recognise the needs of their relative in terms of *when* to support and *when* to encourage independence.

What we do

At the Wolfson, brain injury education and its impact, particularly on communication, is tailored to meet individuals' needs and abilities. With all patients on the SLT caseload we complete baseline outcome measures (unless considered to be clinically inappropriate). One aspect of this is a 'client admission self-report', which proves a useful guide when beginning to ascertain the level of education needed for that individual. The patient is supported to answer questions about their brain injury and what they know about their communication difficulties. This can then be used to guide further exploration and plan the appropriate therapeutic approach.

Individual therapy sessions

At some level, the majority of our patients will have a number of one-to-one sessions with their lead therapist to explore further their understanding of brain injury and communication disability, and to provide them with relevant information. These can range from a one-off session to an ongoing therapeutic process throughout their stay, often supported by the SLT assistant, and will be determined in part by the severity of the patient's communication difficulty. The process allows clients to take on information at their own pace and provides the opportunity for repetition, clarification and feedback and time to ask questions, all within a safe and supportive environment, thus helping clients to understand their communication difficulty and begin to come to terms with the changes.

These sessions may result in the joint compilation of a 'personalised information sheet' or DVD about the person's brain injury and specific communication difficulty (see Figures 9 and 10 on pages 42 and 43). The information sheet may also include strategies and advice to support the individual's communication. The process is a therapy tool, educating and informing the patient and, if involved, family and friends.

The compilation of such an information sheet is encouraged as a joint venture between the patient and the speech and language therapist or assistant to ensure the patient makes choices and to take decisions about what information to include in the information sheet, how much information, and the language and format used.

Importantly, this process will provide the patient with a permanent record and enables self-advocacy and the means to explain their brain injury and communication changes to others. Further one-to-one and group sessions may also be provided to incorporate use of the information sheets in real-life settings and to inform a wider audience, for example when out shopping or when out with friends.

Education groups

Education about brain injury is also carried out in a group setting. A well-recognised and respected aspect of SLT provision at the Wolfson is the Education Group, which takes place over a period of approximately six weeks. This is normally for those patients with less severe communication difficulties and those with cognitive-communication disorder. Each session lasts an hour and takes place once a week. The content of each session is predetermined and set out in a booklet (the *Brain Injury Education Book*, McIntosh & Leach, 2008) that covers each of the six weeks with a specific 'chapter' or topic: for example, the functions of the brain and the mechanism of brain injury; communication difficulties following brain injury; physical difficulties; case studies. The pack becomes the patient's property to take away at the end of the group and there are opportunities and support for individuals to annotate the pack with personal examples and information. While the resource is predetermined, each week's session is tailored and adapted to meet the group's needs. The sessions are interactive and patients are encouraged to share their experiences, ask questions and make comments at all stages of the process.

Members of the SLT team and an SLT student at the Wolfson developed the *Brain Injury Education Book* when it became very apparent that there was a need for such a tool. Over time it has been adapted and amended through consultation with patients who have been through the group to ensure it is meeting the needs of the users. More recently, a patient who was at the Wolfson has been involved in illustrating the book, using his experience of living with aphasia and cognitive-communication disorder. This has been so useful and well received that it has been sponsored and published by Wandsworth PCT Race for Life.

My communication

I have aphasia and apraxia. This is as a result of my stroke.

APHASIA – difficulty understanding and producing spoken and written language
APRAXIA – difficulty organising the sounds and segments in speech

Because of this it is not as easy for me to communicate as it used to be.
I do understand most things. My main problems are with getting my thoughts
across and my speech out clearly.

Things I can do to support my communication

Talk   Write things down

Use gesture and pointing   Use my facial expression

Using a *combination* of these is the most successful way
for me to communicate

Things others can do to support my communication

Write things
down   Check with me that
they have understood
me correctly

Give me choices if they haven't understood what I said,
eg 'Rooney?', 'Rinaldo?'

Figure 9 A personalised information sheet for a man with aphasia and apraxia

What I want to achieve in my conversations

- To be contributing to conversations
- To make a relevant contribution
- To listen well to all points of view
- To be perceived as someone who can make a contribution that is valid
- To be honest in my contributions
- I need to clarify what and how I want to be perceived in a conversation, so that the other person understands the difficulties I sometimes have in achieving the above

I have cognitive-communication difficulties as a consequence of my brain injury. This means my conversation skills are different from how they were before. Through identifying some rules for me and my conversation partner I am able to compensate for some of the difficulties and continue to enjoy RELEVANT, VALID and HONEST conversations.

My rules for conversations

- Avoid external distractions – think about my position
- Avoid internal distractions – try and focus on the speaker
- When I'm distracted I need to 'come back down to earth'
    - Look at   other person
    - Explain I've got lost
    - Ask for a reminder of the topic
- Go a bit slower, don't jump straight in with a comment or answer:
    - ⬤ Stop
    - ◯ Think – 'Is this relevant/valid?'
    - ⬤ Go
- If I find myself in a conversation that is going off track or getting complicated, I need to STOP and ask for help. Don't wing it!

Rules for my conversation partner

- It's important you are not overbearing – don't take over the conversation or talk for me
- You need to keep me on track if things are going astray
- You need to check with me to see if what I am saying is true:
    - Ask a direct question to find out, eg 'Do you actually grow green beans?'
- If what I am saying doesn't make sense, you need to stop me immediately with honest direct feedback:
    - 'Patty, are you sure that's what you mean?'
    - 'Patty, that doesn't make sense'
- If I get distracted you need to remind me of the topic and be firm about bringing me back on track:
    - 'You seem to have got distracted … we were talking about X'

Figure 10 A personalised information sheet for a woman with cognitive-communication difficulties

The Total Communication Group, also run by the SLT department, is for patients with severe aphasia. This group provides them with a safe and supportive environment in which to engage in conversation and practise total communication strategies. The Total Communication Group is often used as an alternative forum in which to provide education about brain injury and aphasia. It enables patients to access information and to increase their understanding at a pace and level that suits them.

Multidisciplinary team working

We work closely with our psychology colleagues, particularly with regard to those individuals with cognitive-communication disorder. Joint sessions to feed back assessment results can begin to raise awareness and insight as a precursor to realistic goal negotiation around communication. Use of shared language and terminology is key to ensuring that the information and education provided are consistent and meaningful for the patient. A motivational counselling approach is often used to help patients move to the next stage of readiness for therapy. The idea of goals is an important component of motivational counselling; clarifying a person's goals and identifying discrepancies between current behaviour and abilities and their desired goals provides the basis for change (Gauggel & Hoop, 2003). For those patients with impaired insight, a relevant goal for their rehabilitation, supported by all members of the multidisciplinary team, may be 'to understand the basic details of my brain injury and its consequences, and to be able to explain this to my family and friends'.

Giving a diagnosis

Where it is identified as useful for a patient and/or their family and friends, we may arrange for patients to see and discuss their brain scans with a doctor. The speech and language therapist will frequently be involved to support communication and understanding. This may indeed be initiated by the patient: as they acquire information about the brain, its function and the effect of damage, patients often want to see the scans for themselves to really see how *their* brain has been injured, to help them put the pieces of the puzzle together. This can prove to be an empowering experience, but one that also needs support as many people find it sparks the sudden realisation that this is long-term condition.

We make use of consistent and recognised terminology during therapy and all parts of the rehabilitation process: in joint sessions, during goal-planning meetings, in discussions with family and friends. We use the term 'brain injury' to emphasise commonalities and reinforce that it is the brain that is affected regardless of the mechanism causing the injury (for example stroke, aneurysm, TBI etc). We also ensure that patients know the terminology that describes the mechanism of their neurological condition, and are able to use it in a way that is meaningful for them.

We use the recognised communication impairment 'labels' (aphasia, cognitive-communication disorder, dyspraxia, dysarthria etc.) to give the individual's difficulty a name and to demystify their experience. We have found that this helps patients (and their families) to recognise changes to their communication and the impact of these changes. Giving the impairment an 'official' label can pave the way for identifying supportive strategies and facilitate the process of adjustment.

Case studies

John's education strand

- Day 1 – given SLT information leaflet about service
- Attended Education Group early in admission (17 October 2007)
- Received *Brain Injury Education Book* with aphasia-friendly design
- Individualised aphasia education using cognitive neuropsychology model
- Joint session with doctors to support understanding of medical information
- Education of family, simplified for children
- Consistent feedback about diagnosis and prognosis (in communication and other areas)

Paolo's education strand

A man of 67 with long-term diagnosis of ataxia, previously misdiagnosed. Acoustic neuroma recently diagnosed and removed – profound facial palsy; uncoordinated swallow. Mild cognitive impairment.

- Paolo and wife had discussion with speech and language therapist regarding nature and history of his swallowing disorder, using diagrams and statistics regarding risks.
- Written information was given to Paolo and wife to read and discuss.
- Doctor and therapist were available for a question/answer session (knowledge of the nature of disorder and risk were discussed).
- Risk assessment, regarding the introduction of small amounts of syrup-consistency food, was carried out and discussed with Paolo, wife and treating team.
- Videofluoroscopy video used with Paolo and wife to demonstrate his swallowing disorder and aspiration.
- Choice and capacity issues were discussed with Paolo and wife, with speech and language therapist and psychologist.
- Demonstrations of oral intake given to wife with verbal explanation to Paolo and wife, relating the swallowing precisely to Paolo's dysphagia.
- Written instructions were given with explanations of normal swallowing patterns to work towards and the compensations Paolo should work on.
- Paolo and wife highly intelligent and very knowledgeable about dysphagia but had long-term mistrust of medical profession due to misdiagnosis. Needed to educate them specifically on breakdown of the normal swallow process, consequences for Paolo and risks of therapy aimed at oral intake.

5 Friends and family

The guiding principles for work with friends and family overlap those described in other areas. However, we cannot emphasise enough the importance of involving family and friends in the process of rehabilitation. We can gather much relevant information about our patients from those who know them best, and we can aim to ensure our therapeutic input is maximised and generalised. Furthermore, we must acknowledge what makes up the real-life situation for our patients and compare this with the artificiality of the therapy environment; including the significant others of those we are treating will help to contextualise what we are trying to achieve. It would also be neglectful to ignore the needs of family and friends themselves as they make their own journey along the rehabilitation pathway; we need to be mindful of support for them as they experience challenges, highs and lows along the way.

Guiding principles

Person-centred

A key point to remember is that, even when working closely with relatives, it is the patient who remains the focus of our input. At times there may be conflict or disagreement within the family and it is important to have established clearly that our role is in advocacy and work with the patient rather than a particular family member.

Goal directed

As in other areas, work with family and friends takes place alongside, and is integral to, the goal-planning process. Relatives are involved to the extent that the patient would like them to be and at times they may suggest specific goal areas that they would like to see addressed in therapy. Their opinion may be sought as to the relative priorities of goals and how realistic they might be in the home environment. Again, it is important to emphasise that although their input is valued, our first responsibility is to the client and we will not be able to offer therapy input if a client is not motivated to achieve a relative's goal. The role of the chairperson in the goal-planning process often involves more direct work with family members as they provide a key link between the Wolfson and home. The speech and language therapist is often identified as the chairperson for patients with communication problems owing to the additional support that they can offer the client in meetings and the family in coming to terms with the communication disability. However, they can also act as chairperson outside their normal caseload. In all cases it is important for the speech and language therapist to bear in mind which role they are acting in and where the boundaries are for that role. For example, when acting as chairperson for a client with severe aphasia whose family are struggling to come to terms with the communication difficulty and appear to have had pre-existing difficulties with one another, there may be separate and distinct roles for SLT, psychology and social work.

Multidisciplinary team working

Another fundamental principle is working alongside the multidisciplinary team with friends and family. Our role can overlap with the input provided by other team members, particularly social workers and psychologists, and we need to ensure that we are not duplicating or contradicting work carried out in other sessions. We may also work alongside friends and family in sessions with the multidisciplinary team, for example providing communication support for the patient in a meeting with their family and the social worker.

Flexible approach

We aim to work flexibly with relatives, trying out a variety of particular approaches and innovative ideas specific to their communication situations. For some clients, a structured approach such as SPPARC (Lock *et al*, 2008) is the most valuable, while for others we have worked out an individual approach: for example, devising conversation rules with the client that are practised in the Wolfson with relevant friends and then on a trip out for lunch or coffee. We approach working with families as a collaboration and advise relatives that the clinician might not always have the answer. Solving communication problems relies on both the clinician's expert knowledge of communication and the family's expert knowledge of that particular patient and their communication style and opportunities.

What we do

In practical terms, there are no specific treatment plans that are routinely offered to relatives as each case is evaluated individually. Below are some of the ways in which relatives and friends are involved in SLT at the Wolfson.

Identifying who to involve

The first stage in involving relatives and friends is to gain an idea of who would be most appropriate to be involved in therapy. Usually, the patient will be able to identify who they would like to attend, but occasionally this may be affected by practical factors such as availability. Attendees might include husband/wife, children/grandchildren, mother/father, grandparents, siblings, more distant relatives, close friends or acquaintances. The speech and language therapist often needs to understand a little about the dynamics within the family to ensure that work with them is handled appropriately and is not embarked on in situations where it would not be appropriate. When patients have communication difficulties it can seem as if the family has a louder voice than the patient. One advantage of the rehabilitation centre setting is that it ensures that the relationship with the patient is the predominant one. The speech and language therapist can therefore have a role as advocate for the patient within their family. It is important that the therapist is aware of their role in difficult situations and ensures that communication remains at the forefront of their involvement in a case.

Information gathering

We gather information from relatives and friends in a number of different ways and for a number of differing purposes. We use both standardised (MCLA, see Appendix) and informal questionnaires, face-to-face discussion and telephone liaison. We want to know about communication styles and opportunities both before and since the brain injury. We also need to know if there are any family circumstances that might be impacting on someone's communication. Concern about where they will live when discharged or the impact of the brain injury on their family may make someone unable to concentrate on their therapy. The speech and language therapist will gather information from friends and family as therapy progresses. Information about the communication environment is assimilated and accumulated gradually.

Home visits

Speech and language therapists can find it difficult to prioritise the need to attend home visits with patients. However, occasionally the information gained from these visits can be invaluable in guiding therapy and for this reason we feel it is sometimes justified to carry out one or two home visits. Sometimes a home visit enables contact with a relative who might otherwise find it difficult to attend therapy sessions. On other occasions, it can facilitate communication around issues relating to the return home, for example, which room a patient might like to sleep in. Sometimes it helps to see a patient communicating in their own environment or using their own things. This adds a different perspective to our understanding of the patient and their communication needs. It also allows us to see how home relates to therapy and, possibly, to establish further goals. We can highlight appropriate topics for conversation or to explore further in a communication folder. In some circumstances it may be appropriate to use a home visit to investigate the local area and identify possible social support or activities.

Education

Just as we believe it is of paramount importance to provide brain injury and communication-related education to patients, it is also important to ensure that those around them are informed too. We provide this education in a number of ways. We use freely available leaflets such as those produced by, for example, the Stroke Association and Speakability alongside those we have devised ourselves. Often patients are involved in creating their own personalised information sheets or communication rules, which can then be shared with those around them. On other occasions we provide education face to face along with direct advice on supporting communication. In some situations, the most appropriate format for providing education is via video and in these cases we might develop a self-advocacy video with the client.

A key way of providing information and advice to relatives is through the Wolfson 'Friends and Family' programme. This is a weekly discussion group advertised widely in the Centre and freely available to all friends and relatives of patients attending. The programme covers four topics: Brain Injury Explained, Physical Changes and Care Needs, Communication after Brain Injury, and Life after the Wolfson. Each session is facilitated by one or two members of the multidisciplinary team and provides both didactic teaching on the topic and opportunities for discussion, questions and peer support.

Expectations

Closely linked to the education of relatives is how we deal with their expectations of therapy. Relatives can at times be very unrealistic in their expectations and find it hard to hear information that does not fit with their current expectations. Soon after the acute hospital admission, many family members may talk in a way that suggests they are on a 'restoration narrative', expecting that their relative can achieve their pre-morbid level of functioning with sufficient therapy input. We try to be aware of both the relatives' and the patient's current level of adjustment and acceptance, and offer support in coming to terms with changes. We need to offer honest, clear information to relatives about our expectations and prognosis but must be aware of whether they are able to take this on board. We make plans for the future given the family's level of adjustment and acceptance. For example, it may not be helpful to provide a communication book for a client with severe aphasia if no one around them is willing to use it.

Support

As part of the education and awareness raising we also provide support to friends and families of patients in dealing with communication change. This may be practical support in terms of strategies they can learn to improve communication, or emotional support in terms of their adjustment to the changes in conversations. Although we can offer support to relatives during the patient's time at the Wolfson, we cannot be involved after discharge and for that reason we encourage people to explore more long-term support options, whether that is through informal support networks or accessing services.

Therapy

There are numerous ways in which friends and family can be included in therapy sessions and their involvement can vary from seeing the therapist in their own right (as in 'Conversation Partner' training programmes) to just sitting in to observe what happens in sessions. A few examples of ways in which relatives might be involved in sessions are given below.

Facilitating communication

Family or friends are often the key conversation partners for the patient and for this reason it is important that they are able to provide the facilitation needed by the patient to ensure meaningful, enjoyable conversations and in order to maintain their relationship. Sometimes this training might follow a prescribed pattern of intervention, such as the conversation partner training offered by the SPPARC programme (Lock *et al*, 2008). On other occasions it might be an informal training session offered by the speech and language therapist, for example introducing how to use a patient's conversation rules. These sessions can take place in a variety of locations including out and about in the community and in the patient's own home.

Carrying out therapy tasks

If the client will benefit from more regular input than can be offered by the SLT department, it may be appropriate to use a relative to carry out some therapy tasks. This works best when the task is repetitive and the friend or relative visits regularly and can be trained in how to support the client in carrying out the task. The therapy task may be dysarthria exercises, word-finding exercises or swallowing exercises, to name but a few. We need to consider the relationship between the client and friend or family member, however, and ensure that this 'teaching' role does not impact on their ability to have other conversations and interactions. Both patient and relative need to be clear when they do, and do not, want to carry out these tasks.

Video interaction

Video interaction work can be a productive way of improving conversations with a key conversation partner. It may follow a specific programme such as SPPARC or be adapted to the particular patient. We use video interaction work with a range of communication diagnoses as it helps both patient and relative to identify goal areas for improvement in their conversations and provides a concrete record of how adaptations to their communication can have an impact on the success of the conversation.

Conclusions

Working with friends and family is a very important strand of our work at the Wolfson, but as with all strands it may be more or less significant for each individual patient. This chapter covers some of the more common ways in which we work in this area, but a key feature is flexibility of working and individualising what is offered both to the patient and to the friends and family who are involved.

Case studies

John's friends and family strand

- Wife involved at pre-admission phase.
- Early telephone liaison with wife.
- Work and family commitments and distance from home to Centre meant liaison with family was often via telephone rather than face to face.
- Wife and John attended regular two-weekly goal-planning meetings with treating team.
- Wife and children attended sessions with speech and language therapist.
- Brother attended 'Friends and Family' education session.
- Speech and language therapist supported chairperson in liaising with family.
- Explored pre-morbid social activities with John to determine need to involve friends.

Patty's friends and family strand

A woman of 47 with cognitive-communication disorder following encephalitis.

- Husband involved at pre-admission phase.
- Speech and language therapist allocated as chairperson.
- Ongoing direct liaison and contact with husband – face to face, telephone and email.
- Husband regularly involved in therapy sessions and initiated arranging additional one-to-one sessions with himself and the speech and language therapist to discuss his involvement and issues in relation to communication.
- Patty and husband attended regular two-weekly goal-planning meetings with treating team.
- Goal relating to conversations with friends identified importance of friends in Patty's life – liaison with friends through husband and by email. Patty and the speech and language therapist made regular community trips to café to meet friends and educate about communication changes and practise use of conversational rules.
- Husband attended 'Friends and Family' education session.
- Ongoing support by email via husband after discharge.

6 Psychosocial adjustment

Rehabilitation cannot be approached without due consideration and time given to the psychosocial adjustment of the patient, their family and/or carers. This key strand makes up a large part of our work with brain-injured patients at the Wolfson as they encounter new challenges, struggles and achievements along their journey, and as they and their significant others begin to come to terms with the changes in their lives and to their identity. It is naïve to think that we can attempt to effectively rehabilitate someone if we fail to acknowledge and begin to address the emotional and psychological consequences that are part and parcel of a life-changing experience.

Just as rehabilitation is a pathway, so too is the process of adjustment. There are no set rules for how we as individuals adjust to something as significant as brain injury. It is the job of the therapist and the multidisciplinary team to treat each patient individually, tailoring their approach to meet the needs of where on the 'adjustment curve' the patient is at a particular time. For example, someone who can tell you about their disorder but is unable to accept it requires a different approach from someone who is well adjusted to their potential future. It is also important to recognise that we are only involved for a snapshot of time on the long-term path that continues for life. It is imperative therefore that we explore and facilitate psychosocial adjustment for the long term.

A simple definition of identity suggests that it is a composite of roles, values and beliefs that are acquired and maintained through social interaction. We project an identity in social interactions by talking and acting in certain ways, and our negotiation of identity is ongoing. Parr *et al* (2001) suggest that with aphasia it is fundamentally social identity that has altered. Communication difficulties may rob the individual of the ability to project themselves effectively. Furthermore, the authors point out that significant others will also experience identity challenges.

Patients may find themselves at a crossroads, with difficult decisions to make as to which path or direction to take. Renegotiating and building identity and adjusting to the new situation can become an obstacle course for all those involved. It is vital that during rehabilitation psychosocial support is available. Identifying the best person to provide the support takes skill and holistic, flexible thinking. Less experienced therapists need to seek guidance from their team in order to provide the most appropriate source. As with all phases and approaches to rehabilitation, flexibility is key.
Often described as invaluable by our patients is the social support that can be gained from others in similar positions, so it may be the expert volunteer or another patient in a conversation group who can provide the support, just as much as any member of the multidisciplinary team.

For people with communication difficulties, the speech and language therapist may play a key role in facilitating the exploration of adjustment. Communication impairment may mean the patient is unable to access other support and some of the more traditional approaches, often described as 'talking therapies', and this may reduce their ability to discuss issues and adjust to the changes occurring for themselves and their families. In essence then, the problem with addressing identity and adjustment challenges in people with communication difficulties is complicated by the words we use to capture the essence of identity (Shadden & Agan, 2004). It is our role then to facilitate and support an individual's communicative competence, be it directly or indirectly, in order to derive maximum benefit from psychosocial approaches.

Guiding principles

At the Wolfson there are core principles that we consider guide the psychosocial adjustment strand of our SLT input. These are uppermost in our minds when we approach goal negotiation and decision making with our patients and their friends and families.

Preparation for discharge – starts from time of arrival

Something that can often come as a shock to patients and their relatives is our focus on discharge from the moment the person arrives at the Wolfson. A discharge date that may seem a long way off to a patient will in all reality come around very quickly. Discharge marks a significant step along the journey and it is essential that we prepare our patient and their families for this next stage.

Appropriate timing

Every patient coming through the Wolfson is seen as and treated as an individual. We cannot be prescriptive in what we do and when we do it, but rather must explore with the patient and their significant others where they are in the process of coming to terms with this phase of their life. This exploration then guides how we support and facilitate psychosocial adjustment.

Exploring

Exploration is a key principle for all the strands of our input, but is perhaps uppermost when we are considering the process of adjustment. We explore areas such as timing denial versus lack of awareness and insight; sense of self before and after brain injury; perception of and reaction to disability; changes to roles and relationships within the family and reactions to them (to name but a few). This exploration is as integral a part of the rehabilitation as specific individualised treatment programmes. LeMay (1993) made the following powerful statement highlighting the link between aphasia and social identity: 'up until the night before the ... [stroke], the person with aphasia was ... an integral part of society, considering himself a lifetime member, without questioning his status. He was society.' Shadden & Agan (2004) acknowledge that, unfortunately, most societies value independence, measure identity in terms of contributions, and reject illness and impairment. Being aware of this is key when we are exploring personal constructs with our patients: that person was society and therefore they may hold those same views and will need to be well supported in the renegotiation of identity.

Facilitation

Facilitating psychosocial adjustment forms a basis of the rehabilitation process for all members of the multidisciplinary team when they are working with patients at the Wolfson. It is acknowledged that people with aphasia are especially vulnerable to issues of identity change (Kagan & Duchan, 2004; Lapointe, 2001; Shadden, 2005). However, the presence of aphasia has implications for the ability to work through these issues via language, as other individuals would (Armstrong & Ulatowska, 2007). Particularly for those patients with communication disability then, the speech and language therapist is required to play a key facilitative role, using specialist skills to support those for whom traditional 'talking therapies' may not be appropriate. This may be done in individual sessions or jointly with other members of the team as and when issues and concerns arise. It is also of vital importance that we share relevant facilitative communication techniques with our colleagues so that adjustment can be further supported throughout the rehabilitation journey, and those techniques are specifically tailored to the individual.

Education

Person-centred education about brain injury and its consequences, particularly in relation to communication disability, should form a foundation layer of input if we are to successfully support the patient and their family in living with their communication disability. It is not enough to assume that those involved have been given information about their condition and what to expect; literature suggests that people need to be given such information at least three to four times before they start to take it on board and accept it. Therefore ongoing exploration and provision of information has to be integral in our daily contact with patients and their families as and when the need arises.

Working with family and friends

Family and/or friends play a key role in adjustment, yet as we discuss in the 'Friends and Family' strand, the focus of our input must remain the patient. It is wrong, however, to ignore the psychosocial needs of those closely involved with the patient, and we must find appropriate ways to support them in coming to terms with the change in their family member or friend and the issues this may raise for them. Furthermore, as we have already identified, the therapist is only involved for a snapshot of time along the journey and it is those who will be around the patient for the long term who will ultimately 'live with' the condition alongside the patient. Working together can aim to ensure that all involved are 'living with' the condition rather than suffering because of it (McIntosh, 2008).

Promoting self-help

A guiding principle must be to encourage the patient and those around them not to become dependent on the therapist as the support provision. We must be mindful of the fact that therapy comes to an end (often earlier than we would like owing to service constraints) and so we should be exploring with our patients, even in the early days, how they can help themselves.

Raising insight

For patients with cognitive impairment a lack of insight impedes the process of adjustment. How can someone begin to adjust to change or a difficulty if they do not see that the change or difficulty exists? Education and supportive feedback informs the insight-raising process and must be done in a way that is constructive and therapeutic for all those involved. Consideration of Prochaska & Diclemente's 'wheel of change' (1986), originally devised for their work within complex health behaviours and change, can provide us with a useful guide when exploring an individual's readiness and motivation to change. It can guide clinical decisions about what to offer, where and when, and helps to identify what our role is at that time. It is important to match what we offer with the stage the client is at: should we be information providers to help with insight, or should intervention be more active once insight starts to emerge?

Six stages of the wheel of change

1 Precontemplation – lack of awareness that life can be improved by a change in behaviour

2 Contemplation – recognition of the problem, initial consideration of behaviour change, and information gathering about possible solutions and actions

3 Preparation – introspection about the decision, reaffirmation of the need and desire to change behaviour, and completion of final pre-action steps

4 Action – implementation of the practices needed for successful behaviour change

5 Maintenance – consolidation of the behaviours initiated during the action stage

6 Termination – former problem behaviours are no longer perceived as desirable

Adapted from Prochaska & Diclemente, 1986

Group support

Over the years, group interventions have been identified as vehicles for addressing some of the broader psychosocial challenges of aphasia (Avent, 1997; Elman, 1999; Marshall, 1999). At the Wolfson we see this as applying not only to aphasia, but to all communication impairments, and have found that groups can be a powerful tool in terms of support and adjustment. A therapist may be an expert in the nature of communication disability and how best to support an individual, but they cannot be an expert in what it is like to experience and live with the changes that accompany an acquired disability. This is the challenge facing both the patient and their family and friends. The group itself can provide a social space for dealing with personal issues, opening the door to identity validation. Group support is a key principle that influences the support we offer and how we offer it.

Supporting transition to community: inreach and outreach

This principle runs alongside those of timing and preparation for discharge. At the Wolfson we recognise that, due to the nature of our service, we can currently only offer short-term support for adjustment, and that because of this we may only have started 'tapping the surface' of the process for those involved. The *National Service Framework for Long-term Conditions* (Department of Health, 2005) recommends a model that meets the continuing and changing needs through provision of rehabilitation, advice and support. To fulfil this requires person-centred input that includes social reintegration, adjustment and long-term support. We can facilitate this long-term provision by working with our colleagues in the community, ensuring close and, where possible, joint working, continuation of goal setting and transparency of transition for the patient and their family.

What we do

The individual nature of psychosocial adjustment means that there can be no one specific or prescribed treatment plan that we hand out to patients as they walk through the doors of the Wolfson.
We outline below techniques that we use regularly and have found to be successful, adapting them to the individual in order to begin facilitating and supporting the process of adjustment for our patients with communication disability.

Insight raising

This starts from the assessment stage. Regular feedback of assessment results, both formal and informal, is a good starting point. In addition to language and communication assessments, we use tools such as BICRO-39; S24; VASES; CAPCI (see Appendix for further details of these tools); self-reports; family questionnaires; video baseline and self-evaluation; personalised rating scales. These provide valuable information for us, but perhaps more importantly they can help frame for the individual how their communication disability is impacting or will impact on their life and so begin the process of adjustment. Ongoing use of video evaluation (for example, videos made with therapists, with family members, in multidisciplinary team sessions) and education for the patient and their family and friends throughout therapy continues to raise insight and help the patient come to terms with the difficulties and changes they are experiencing.

Advocacy

We provide our patients with advocacy support and promote self-advocacy in a number of ways.
Goal planning is at the core of rehabilitation at the Wolfson, but the goal-planning meetings (and

indeed other meetings that may be necessary, such as case conferences, meetings with carers) may be overwhelming or 'scary' for a patient with communication difficulties. We provide support by talking about forthcoming meetings and identifying key issues the patient may want to raise in addition to goal areas. Use of appropriate total communication (TC) strategies can then be taught to all those involved and used during the meetings to facilitate the patient's involvement and ensure that they have their say.

Provision of 'I've had a stroke/brain injury' cards and support to use them in real-life situations can help as people start to reintegrate into the community. These might be ready-made (for example, those provided by the Stroke Association that fit into a wallet) or tailor-made (for example, in therapy sessions used to personally design information leaflets or cards about communication difficulties and ways to support communication). They can also be produced in DVD format, which is particularly useful when there will be carers involved, for example, at a nursing or residential home. Developing such information in an educational way serves to empower the patient as they then own their communication disability and can inform others about it and how best to help them.

Working with family and friends

As discussed, family and friends play a key role in psychosocial adjustment, and indeed bring their own adjustment issues to the rehabilitation process. Simply inviting family and friends to therapy sessions and involving them informally in our therapy can be a powerful tool in overcoming fears and concerns they may have in dealing with communication difficulties. This can build confidence in the use of communication strategies and help them see how best to support communication and interactions between them and the patient.

We aim to provide opportunities to talk together about the changes and difficulties family and friends are experiencing; this can be a useful experience for all involved and the use of supportive counselling skills is vital. Use of video can be very helpful here, identifying together the changes, what strategies help communication and the barriers that may be experienced. We often make use of a SPPARC type approach (Lock *et al*, 2008) at varying levels, depending on relevance and appropriateness, and video conversations between the patient and someone they have identified, taking the therapist out of the situation in order to facilitate a more normal, real-life interaction. These are then evaluated together in further sessions. Opportunities for conversation practice and making use of information sheets (for example, agreed conversation rules devised for the patient and their conversation partner) can support the process of change and adjustment. We have done this in a variety of settings and have found them most valuable when used to support transition into the community (for example, meeting a friend for coffee in a café).

Giving family and friends their own time is also important. At the Wolfson we run a 'Friends and Family' group on a weekly basis. This is time for family and friends without the patients present. Each session has a particular topic, but the programme is intended to be a number of informative, supportive sessions where people can ask questions, gather information and, perhaps more importantly, share experiences with fellow families and friends, adopting the idea of themselves as experts in their situation.

Education

We provide education in one-to-one and group sessions, with individuals and with family and friends, depending on what is most appropriate. Sessions occur regularly where we inform about brain function and what happens when damage occurs, and provide specific details about the communication disorder. These sessions often then form the basis of personalised information sheets (see Chapter 4 'Education'). We also run a weekly education group where patients with varying disorders follow an education book (McIntosh & Leach, 2008) covering a variety of topics (this is covered in more depth in Chapter 4). We find there is great value in this environment as people begin to share their experiences and learn from one another, helping the process of adjustment.

We also see our role as supporting the patient to gather information from other sources: for example, facilitating a session with the doctor to look at the patient's brain scan or discuss concerns, medication etc. This can be very useful in helping the person understand the medical side of their condition and can support them in comprehending the irreversible or long-term damage that has occurred. Doing so can help to move the patient from a curative narrative to a quest narrative (Kleinman, 1998).

Confidence building

Key to helping someone adjust to the changes they are experiencing is building confidence in their new ways of communicating and their new role. We recognise confidence-based goals as a valid reason for SLT input and create situations where people can try out their skills and techniques in a safe environment – for example one-to-one sessions, small group sessions, role play, sessions with family, telephone use – before they try things out in the community. We have encouraged and supported patients to take a chairing or facilitative role in a group they have been attending where this has been a goal negotiated. Joint sessions with other members of the multidisciplinary team can also serve to build confidence in communication skills: for example, a shopping trip with occupational and speech and language therapists, visiting the gym with physio- and speech and language therapists, visiting the office to see a manager or old colleagues, exploring voluntary work options at the local volunteer bureau, to mention just a few examples. To measure confidence we make use of personalised rating scales and employ video to help patients evaluate themselves (see Figure 11).

Linking with support groups

We encourage patients and their family to explore support groups, particularly for longer-term support and adjustment. Again, this may be done in individual sessions, using telephone directories and the internet, or through groups such as Education Group and Friends and Family sessions. These activities may be followed up by us accompanying the patient on a visit to the support group or day centre, or facilitating this opportunity with another key person. The American Stroke Association's website has described the support group as 'a community organisation for stroke survivors and their family members, friends and others. It helps people learn more about their stroke, share their experiences about stroke, and become inspired to move forward after their stroke'. Recognition of the value of such organisations is an important facet of our work.

Use of expert volunteers

We are very fortunate that we have two regular volunteers working in the SLT department. Both are former patients with aphasia and we have found them invaluable in the supportive role they can provide to current patients. We make use of their 'expert skills' in various ways: they tell current patients their stories, listen to the patients' stories and demonstrate their own use of TC strategies. Patients have reported benefit in terms of adjustment through seeing someone who is further along the journey. It is important to recognise, however, that this is not found to be helpful by everyone and involving a volunteer needs to be thought through case by case. Some patients may feel it is too early to see someone 'at the next stage' and indeed may be scared and overwhelmed by this exposure. Others may find it counterproductive in terms of motivation and insight. Timing and readiness are key principles to consider.

CONVERSATION RATING SCALES

Completed by: **Date:**

1 In conversation I produce my words accurately

Never	Occasionally	Sometimes	Frequently	Always
1	2	3	4	5

2 In conversation there are long pauses while I think of a word

Never	Occasionally	Sometimes	Frequently	Always
1	2	3	4	5

3 In conversation, when I offer my opinion/ideas it is a useful contribution

Never	Occasionally	Sometimes	Frequently	Always
1	2	3	4	5

4 I am an integral part of family decision making

Never	Occasionally	Sometimes	Frequently	Always
1	2	3	4	5

5 I can support C in talking to the children sensitively and appropriately

Never	Occasionally	Sometimes	Frequently	Always
1	2	3	4	5

Figure 11 A personalised rating scale for conversation developed with John

Video evaluation: pre and post therapy

Using video before therapy commences and again towards the end of therapy is a great outcome measure and can be very helpful for adjustment. It is difficult to identify change and progress on a daily basis, and stepping outside of therapy can be a challenge for all those involved. Video use should be approached with care, however, as something we may view as progress in terms of therapy may not be viewed in the same way by the patient. Using a semi-structured approach such as focusing on key communication aspects or parameters, and making use of pre and post rating scales can help support this process. Encouraging open discussion and feedback can aid the therapist in identifying areas that need further exploration and support, perhaps at the next stage of rehabilitation.

Use of counselling skills: working with neuropsychology and neuropsychiatry

It is recognised that sense of self and self-esteem can be profoundly impacted on when someone's means of communication is altered. While we have specialist skills in communication therapy and make use of counselling skills in much of what we do at the Wolfson, it is imperative that we work closely with our psychology and psychiatry colleagues, particularly when we feel psychosocial issues arise that are beyond our expertise. By putting multidisciplinary team working and goal planning at the core of our approach at the Wolfson we are able to negotiate joint goals with the psychology department and address these accordingly. This may be through joint one-to-one sessions and joint family sessions, or it may be to support the patient's communication during psychology/neuropsychiatry sessions. It is also important to recognise changes in mood, particularly as insight improves, and it may be necessary to refer to our colleagues for assessment and advice. This extends to family and friends, being mindful of how they are moving along the process of adjustment and that they may need a more specific counselling approach that we are unable to offer. Prompt and timely referral is therefore key.

Group support and the importance of narrative

As mentioned, fellow patients and the 'expert patient' model provide a very valuable source of support for adjustment. We run a range of groups at the Wolfson (for example Lost for Words, Loud and Clear, Conversation Group, Education Group, Total Communication, Assertiveness Group, Out and About) all of which incorporate the opportunity to share and learn from one another. Regardless of severity, it seems a great deal can be gained from seeing another person in a similar situation manage to communicate thoughts and feelings in whatever way they can. Similarly, hearing someone tell their story can be a very powerful and beneficial experience. Rowe (2004) highlights that stories, or autobiographical narratives, are the primary means through which we create meaning and purpose in our lives, and the structure of stories is one of the key organising principles that brings order to the complexity of our experiences. He describes writer and editor Robert McCrum, who at 42 had a severe stroke. Reflecting in his book *My Year Off: Rediscovering Life After a Stroke* (1998), written some years later, McCrum acknowledged that writing the book served his need to make sense of his experiences and the huge changes in his life.

The therapist can play a key role within the group, for example by facilitating those with more impaired communication. Taking a more specific therapeutic role may also be appropriate (perhaps in individual sessions) to help an individual explore their own narrative and, if appropriate, gradually help them change their story or 'recast themselves' within it so their story is no longer as 'toxic' or damaging as it may have been.

Out and about

This part of therapy has been referred to previously, but it is deserving of a special mention as 'Out and About' forms a big part of our therapy provision at the Wolfson. We view getting out into the community as a very worthwhile and, where possible, essential part of our therapy. Accompanying individuals and groups on trips – to the shops, pub, post office, library, garden centre, for example – regularly occurs when directed by the goals negotiated. This can support confidence and the use of communication and/or swallowing strategies, and help overcome the stigma that patients may be feeling about themselves, as well as enabling them to see that there can be a future ahead, thus supporting the process of change.

Building new self and reconstruction of identity

We have learned much from Ylvisaker et al's (2008) approach, using the idea of metaphor, role models and a person's own constructs in order to support our patients in the difficult area of reconstruction of identity. As professionals working in the rehabilitation field, we are familiar and, hopefully, comfortable with disability; however, a patient going through the rehabilitation process as the person with disability may be experiencing a mix of emotions about how it feels to be disabled. Thinking about the future, acknowledging a possible loss of role and the task of reconstructing identity can be very daunting. We regularly make use of a 'role model' (for example, Clint Eastwood – Ylvisaker & Feeney, 2000b) and 'metaphor' approach (for example, requests for clarification as journalistic behaviour – Ylvisaker et al, 2008) to help patients unpick how they see themselves in the future and support the process of adjustment and change.

Additional useful approaches include those from personal construct psychology, such as lifestyle grids, dependency grids, support pyramids and self-characterisation.

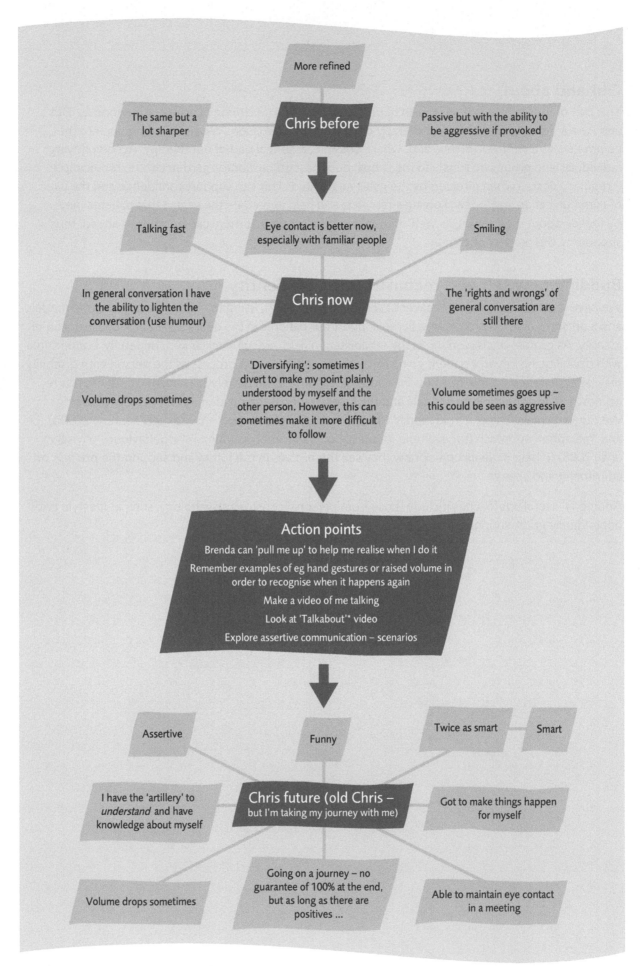

Figure 12 Example of rebuilding identity

* Alex Kelly (2006) *Talkabout* DVD, published by Speechmark Publishing Ltd

Preparing for the next stage of the journey: outreach

Talking openly about discharge and the future from the moment of admission can help to reduce how overwhelmed individuals may feel about the future. We try to make contact with our community team colleagues as early as possible during the admission, although we recognise that this can be difficult owing to service constraints. Inviting a member of the community team to goal-planning meetings has proved useful in the effective handover of information, but perhaps more importantly in helping to prepare the patient and family for what may be in store at the next stage. Knowing that they will be seeing a familiar face, or at least someone they have already met, after discharge can help to support transition. Where possible, we conduct a joint session with a community colleague (often in the patient's home or community) to support the patient in talking about future goals and giving relevant information about themselves. Again, this can be beneficial for empowerment and ownership of goals.

Conclusions

The importance of the psychosocial adjustment strand in rehabilitation should not be underestimated. It is key in ascertaining a patient's readiness for change and therefore our decision making in how we approach their therapy. As with all the strands of rehabilitation, how much we focus on this area will be patient-led, and it may vary at different stages in the rehabilitation journey. A flexible way of working is essential, avoiding being prescriptive in our approach. Listening to the needs of our patients and their family and friends must sit alongside our clinical expertise, and it is important that we balance psychosocial adjustment with the other strands of rehabilitation in order to provide the most appropriate management plan for each individual.

Case studies

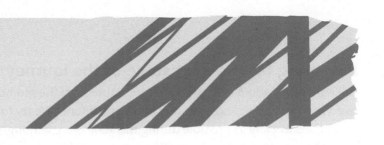

John's psychosocial strand

- John had difficulty accepting aphasia diagnosis and prognosis
- Meeting SLT volunteer with long-term language impairment
- Opportunity for peer support and sharing 'stories' in Brain Injury Education Group
- Developing use of strategies to reduce frustration during conversation
- Use of rating scales to compare a report by the patient with one by his wife and thus adjust perception of difficulties
- Supporting role within family through joint session with wife and children
- Psychosocial support for family, eg Friends and Family meeting – a chance to discuss difficulties in confidence

Sarah's psychosocial strand

A woman of 21 with cognitive-communication disorder and facial weakness following repeated neurosurgery to debulk pineocytoma (brain tumour).

- Developing insight and acceptance regarding higher-level language
- Sarah had lost contact with all her friends – began to discuss new/alternative social opportunities, eg cinema trip with speech and language therapist/groups with other young people
- Exploring and rebuilding self-identity – pre brain injury, now and ideals for the future
- Sarah had reduced self-image/confidence – began to discuss going to hairdresser, new clothes etc.
- Sessions with mum and around mother–daughter relationship – encouraging mum to give back more independence
- Conversation reminder cards for Sarah and her mum to encourage Sarah to take control
- Exploring voluntary work and joint visit with speech and language therapist to volunteer bureau to raise confidence
- Psychological support for Sarah and her family

7 Conclusions

This book has evolved from our passion for working with long-term communication disability and our desire to share with our colleagues our ideas and experiences in neurorehabilitation. It draws on both old and new literature and evidence-based practice in order to provide a reference and a working tool for those involved in this often challenging but exciting field.

Studies show that multidisciplinary rehabilitation is beneficial to patients with brain injury. The Department of Health is now, perhaps more than ever, recognising the importance and value of specialist rehabilitation for people living with brain injury (Healthcare for London, 2009). The long-term cost effectiveness of services is seen alongside the importance of the impact on the patient's journey and their experience. Level of dependency is being considered from a cost point of view and also from a psychosocial standpoint, acknowledging the responsibility of service provision in maximising a person's quality of life and ability to engage in society and chosen lifestyle. The quality of life and issues of family and carers are also being considered.

We cannot therefore emphasise enough the importance of a holistic, client-centred 'life' approach to therapy that spans the services. *Communicating Quality 3* describes the role of the speech and language therapist in aphasia:

> Meeting the needs of individuals with aphasia in maximising their potential for recovery of language, and in developing effective conversation strategies that can be used by both the individual and those they converse with, thereby maintaining their ability to influence their environment, maintain social relationships and quality of life.

> (RCSLT, 2006, p263)

Broaden this to encompass the range of acquired communication disorders that we encounter and you have the basis of SLT provision in neurorehabilitation. Key is the reference to 'life': thinking beyond our therapy bubble and putting everything we do into the context of the patients' journey through their brain injury.

John's comments on his experiences of therapy across settings highlight an important aspect of providing long-term neurorehabilitation:

> The Wolfson is an oasis in a desert. It's a problem for the linking of the things. The woman [community speech and language therapist] is fantastic, absolutely brilliant but the gap is bad. It's very depressing. There's something about the intensity that it's actually doing the brain pathways. That is important.

Although services are arranged along pathways, perhaps attention to transition from one stage of the pathway to the next has been neglected. Gaps need to be filled if we are to put the person at the centre rather than the service. We see each client's journey through his or her brain injury as a long scarf made up of strands. The strands depict the aspects that make up the plan for therapy, and we have found that there are themes for these strands. No one strand is more important than another when we consider the scarf as a whole, but at certain times on the journey one colour may be more prominent than another, as some aspects become more of a priority. However, over time each strand or colour should be represented. The client's stay at the rehabilitation centre is just one small part of the longer scarf, and so the strands we work on should be considered in the light of what comes before, in the acute stage, and after, in community therapy.

Reflecting on the strands at regular intervals during a person's rehabilitation at the Wolfson reminds us of our and the patient's priorities and also what is achievable and realistic at a particular time. Too often we have felt overwhelmed in therapy as we try to address everything at once, perhaps losing sight of the key priorities, the common goals. By being explicit about the strands in case discussions, and regularly and supportively questioning one another in caseload-planning meetings, we have, we believe, become better at looking at the bigger picture. The pressure to 'deal with everything' is reduced as we reflect on the stage of the pathway; the patient's goals and the priority strands that we have agreed with the patient need to be addressed at that time.

By sharing our experiences and evidence with such a 'strands' approach, we may help to develop consistency across services, making transition and the patient's experience more positive and seamless.

John's comments on the strands:

> It is better for the mind to do four things well than actually doing six not very well. But they are all big things, they are all good and important. It's better to do two, then another two, when there is not much time.

Acute hospital

Community therapy and beyond ...

Appendix

Formal and informal assessments available in the Wolfson SLT Department

Admission & Discharge Self Report/Outcome Measure, questionnaire devised by the Wolfson Neurorehabilitation Centre SLT Department for departmental use only.

Aphasia Screening Test, Whurr R (1996) Whurr Publishers, London.

Apraxia Battery for Adults, Dabul B (2000) 2nd edn, Pro-Ed Inc, Austin, TX.

Assessment of Language Related Functional Activities (ALFA) Baines K, Martin A & McMartin Heeringa H (1999) Pro-Ed Inc, Austin, TX.

Boston Naming Test, Kaplan E, Goodglass H & Weintraub S (2000) Lippincott Williams & Wilkins Publishers UK, London.

Brain Injury Community Rehabilitation Outcome Scales (BICRO-39), Powell JH, Beckers K & Greenwood RJ (1998) 'Measuring progress and outcome in community rehabilitation after brain injury with a new assessment instrument – the BICRO-39 scales', *Archives of Physical Medicine and Rehabilitation*, 79 (10), pp1213–25.

Comprehensive Aphasia Test (CAT), Swinburn K, Porter G & Howard D (2004) Psychology Press, Hove, E Sussex.

Conversation Analysis Profile for People with Aphasia (CAPPA), Whitworth A, Perkins L & Lesser R (1997) Whurr Publishers, London.

Conversation Analysis Profile for People with Cognitive Impairment (CAPCI) Perkins L, Whitworth A & Lesser R (1997) Whurr Publishers, London.

Dysarthria Profile, Robertson SJ (1987) Communication Skills Builders Inc, Tucson, AZ.

Erickson S24 Scale, Andrews G & Cutler J (1974) 'S-24 scale. Stuttering therapy: the relations between changes in symptom level and attitudes', *Journal of Speech and Hearing Disorders*, 39, pp312–19.

Frenchay Dysarthria Assessment, Enderby P & Palmer R (2008) 2nd edn, Pro-Ed Inc, Austin, TX.

Low Level Communication Checklist, developed by the Wolfson Neurohabilitation Centre SLT Department for departmental and Centre use.

Measure of Cognitive Linguistic Abilities (MCLA), Ellmo W & Graser J (1995) Speech Bin, Vero Beach, FL.

Mount Wilga High Level Language Test, Christie J, Clark W & Mortensen L (1986), revised Simpson F (2006) unpublished but widely available.

Psycholinguistic Assessments of Language Processing in Aphasia (PALPA) Kay J, Lesser R & Coltheart M (1992) Laurence Erlbaum Associates, Hove, E Sussex.

Relationships and Conversations Questionnaire, devised by the Wolfson Rehabilitation Centre SLT Department, unpublished.

The Autobiographical Memory Interview (AMI), Kopelman M, Baddeley A & Wilson B (1990) Pearson Assessment/PsychCorp, London.

The Awareness of Social Inference Test (TASIT) Flanagan S, McDonald S & Rollins J (2002) Pearson Assessment/PsychCorp, London.

Visual Analogue Self Esteem Scale (VASES) Brumfitt S & Sheeran P (1999) Speechmark Publishing, Milton Keynes.

Computer software

React2, Mitchell P, Runciman L & Allcock D (2008) Propeller Multimedia Ltd, Peebles, UK, www.propeller.net

Speech Sounds on Cue, Bishop C (2004) Propeller Multimedia Ltd, Peebles, UK www.propeller.net

StepbyStep Words, Steps Consulting Ltd (2005) Acton Turville, Sth Glos, www.steps.eu.com

Resources

Brain Injury Education Book, McIntosh J & Leach B (2008) funded by Wandsworth PCT Race for Life, available from The Wolfson Neurorehabilitation Centre.

Charing Cross Assistive Communication Service, Speech & Language Therapy, 2nd Floor North, Charing Cross Hospital, Fulham Palace Road, London W6 8RF, tel. 0208 846 7610.

References

Armstrong E & Ulatowska H (2007) 'Making stories: evaluative language and the aphasia experience', *Aphasiology*, 21 (6/7/8/), pp763–74.

Avent JR (1997) *Manual of Cooperative Group Treatment for Aphasia*, Butterworth-Heinemann, London.

Basso A (2005) 'How intensive/prolonged should an intensive/prolonged treatment be?', *Aphasiology*, 19 (10/11), pp975–84.

Bernier MJ (1993) 'Developing and evaluating printed education materials: a prescriptive model for quality', *Orthopaedic Nursing*, 12, pp39–46.

Bhogal S, Teasell R & Speechley M (2003) 'Intensity of aphasia therapy, impact on recovery', *Stroke*, 34, pp987–93.

Bishop C (2004) *Speech Sounds on Cue*, Propeller Multimedia Ltd, Peebles, UK.

Brady M, Mackenzie C & Armstrong L (2003) 'Topic use following right hemisphere brain damage during three semi-structured conversational discourse samples', *Aphasiology*, 17 (9), pp881–904.

Code C & Muller D (1989) *Aphasia Therapy*, 2nd edn, Cole & Whurr, London.

Department of Health (2001) *The National Service Framework for Older People*, London.

Department of Health (2005) *The National Service Framework for Long-term Conditions*, London.

Department of Health (2007) *A New Ambition for Stroke: A Consultation on a National Strategy*, London.

Ellis EW & Young AW (1998) *Human Cognitive Neuropsychology*, Lawrence Erlbaum Associates, Hove, E Sussex.

Elman RJ (1999) 'Introduction to group treatment of neurogenic communication disorders', Elman RJ (ed), *Group Treatment of Neurogenic Communication Disorders: The Expert Clinician's Approach*, Butterworth-Heinemann, Boston, MA.

Enderby PM, John A & Petheram B (2006) *Therapy Outcome Measures for Rehabilitation Professionals: Speech and Language Therapy, Physiotherapy, Occupational Therapy*, 2nd edn, John Wiley, Chichester.

Frankel T, Penn C & Ormond-Brown D (2007) 'Executive dysfunction as an explanatory basis for conversation symptoms of aphasia: a pilot study', *Aphasiology*, 21 (6–8), pp814–28.

Gauggel S & Hoop M (2003) 'Goal-setting as a motivational technique for neurorehabilitation', Cox W & Klinger E (eds) (2004), *Handbook of Motivational Counseling*, J Wiley, Chichester.

Healthcare for London (2009) *Stroke Rehabilitation Guide: Supporting London Commissioners to Commission Quality Services in 2010/11*, NHS (Commissioning Support for London), London.

Hoffman T, McKenna K, Worrall L & Read S (2004) 'Evaluating current practice in the provision of written information to stroke patients and their carers', *International Journal of Therapy and Rehabilitation*, 11, pp303–9.

James K & Charles N (2008) 'Oiling the wheels of conversation', *RCSLT Bulletin*, 670, pp18–20.

Jones F (2008) 'Stepping out: a programme focusing on self-management after stroke', *International Journal of Therapy and Rehabilitation*, 15 (12), pp540–1.

Kagan A & Duchan JF (2004) 'Consumers' views of what makes therapy worthwhile', Duchan JF & Byng S (eds), *Challenging Aphasia Therapies: Broadening the Discourse and Extending the Boundaries*, Psychology Press, Hove, E Sussex.

Kagan A, Simmons-Mackie N, Rowland A, Huijbregts M, Shumway E, McEwen S, Threats T & Sharp S (2008) 'Counting what counts: a framework for capturing real life outcomes of aphasia intervention', *Aphasiology*, 22 (3), pp258–80.

Kelly A (2005) *Talkabout: A Social Communication Skills Package*, Speechmark Publishing, Milton Keynes (first published 1996 by Winslow).

Kennedy M & Murdoch BE (1994) 'Thalamic aphasia and striato-capsular aphasia as independent aphasic syndromes: a review', *Aphasiology*, 8 (4), pp303–13.

Kiresuk T, Smith A & Cardillo J (eds) (1994) *Goal Attainment Scaling: Applications, Theory and Measurement*, Lawrence Erlbaum Associates, Hillsdale, NJ.

Kleinman A (1998) *The Illness Narratives*, Basic Books, New York.

Lapointe L (2001) 'Darley and the psychosocial side', *Aphasiology*, 15 (3), pp249–60.

LeMay M-A (1993) 'The person with aphasia and society', Lafond D, DeGiovani R, Joanette Y, Ponzio J, Sarno MT, Jarema G & Sherman K (eds), *Living with Aphasia: Psychosocial Issues*, Singular, San Diego, CA.

Lock S, Wilkinson R & Bryan K (2008) *SPPARC: Supporting Partners of People with Aphasia in Relationships & Conversation*, 2nd edn, Speechmark Publishing, Milton Keynes.

Malec J (1999) 'Goal attainment scaling in rehabilitation', Fleminger S & Powell J (eds), *Evaluation of Outcomes in Brain Injury Rehabilitation*, Psychology Press, Hove, East Sussex.

Marshall RC (1999) *Introduction to Group Treatment for Aphasia: Design and Management*, Butterworth-Heinemann, Boston, MA.

McCrum R (1998) *My Year Off: Recovering Life After a Stroke*, Picador, London.

McIntosh J (2008) 'Multidisciplinary neurorehabilitation on chorea-acanthocytosis: a case study', Walker RH, Saiki S & Danek A (eds), *Neuroacanthocytosis Syndromes II*, Springer, Berlin, Heidelberg.

McIntosh J & Leach B (2008) *Brain Injury Education Book*, Wandsworth PCT Race for Life, London.

McIntosh J, Charles N, Cloud G & Rich P (2010) 'Investigating the incidence of cognitive-communication disorder in stroke patients: relating cognitive-communication disorder to site of lesion', poster presentation at 19th European Stroke Conference, Barcelona, and abstract in *Cerebrovascular Diseases*, 29 (suppl 2).

McIntosh J, Lyons B, Charles N & James K (in press) 'Demonstrating change in SLT in neurorehabilitation: it works and patients say it works.'

Milman LH, Holland A, Kaszniak AW, D'Agostino J, Garrett M & Rapcsak S (2008) 'Initial validity and reliability of the SCCAN: using tailored testing to assess adult cognition and communication', *Journal of Speech, Language and Hearing Research*, 51, pp49–69.

Mitchell P, Runciman L & Allcock D (2008) *React2*, Propeller Multimedia Ltd, Peebles, UK.

Orchard CA, Curran V & Kabene S (2005) 'Creating a culture for interdisciplinary collaborative professional practice', *Medical Education Online*, 10 (11), pp1–13.

Paquier PF & Mariën P (2005) 'A synthesis of the role of the cerebellum in cognition', *Aphasiology*, 19 (1), pp3–19.

Parr S, Duchan J & Pound C (1997) *Aphasia Inside Out*, Open University Press, Buckingham.

Parr S, Byng S, Gilpin S & Ireland C (2001) *Talking about Aphasia: Living with the Loss of Language after Stroke*, Open University Press, Buckingham.

Prochaska J & Diclemente C (1986) 'Towards a comprehensive model of change', Miller W & Heather N (eds), *Treating Addictive Behaviors: Processes of Change*, Plenum Press, New York.

Robinson-Smith G, Johnston M & Allen J (2000) 'Self-care self-efficacy, quality of life, and depression after stroke', *Archives of Physical Medicine and Rehabilitation*, 81 (4), pp460–5.

Rowe N (2004) 'We live by the stories we tell: narrative and health', *Therapy Weekly*, December, pp9–12.

RCSLT (Royal College of Speech & Language Therapists) (2006) *Communicating Quality 3*, London.

Royal College of Physicians & British Society of Rehabilitation Medicine (2003) *Rehabilitation Following Acquired Brain Injury: National Clinical Guidelines*, Turner-Stokes L (ed), RCP/BSRM, London.

Schlosser R (2003) 'Goal attainment scaling as a clinical measurement technique in communication disorders: a critical review', *Journal of Communication Disorders*, 37 (3), pp217–39.

Shadden B (2005) 'Aphasia as identity theft: theory and practice', *Aphasiology*, 19 (3/4/5), pp211–23.

Shadden B & Agan J (2004) 'Renegotiation of identity: the social context of aphasia support groups', *Topics in Language Disorders*, 24 (3), pp174–86.

Steps Consulting Ltd (2005) *StepByStep Words*, Acton Turville, Sth Glos, www.steps.eu.com

Turner-Stokes L, Nair A, Sedki I, Disler PB & Wade DT (2009) 'Multi-disciplinary rehabilitation for acquired brain injury in adults of working age', *Cochrane Database of Systematic Reviews 2008*, Issue 3, pp1–44.

World Health Organization (2002) *Towards a Common Language for Functioning, Disability and Health: ICF*, Geneva.

Worrall L, Rose T, Howe T, Brennan A, Egan J, Oxenham D & McKenna K (2005) 'Access to written information for people with aphasia', *Aphasiology*, 19 (10/11), pp923–9.

Ylvisaker M & Feeney T (2000a) 'Reflections on Dobermans, poodles, and social rehabilitation for difficult-to-serve individuals with traumatic brain injury', *Aphasiology*, 14 (4), pp407–32.

Ylvisaker M & Feeney T (2000b) 'Construction of identity after traumatic brain injury', *Brain Impairment*, 1, pp12–28.

Ylvisaker M, McPherson K, Kayes N & Pellett E (2008) 'Metaphoric identity mapping: facilitating goal setting and engagement in rehabilitation after traumatic brain injury', *Neuropsychological Rehabilitation*, 18 (5), pp713–41.